Journey
Beyond
Diagnosis

*Support During and After Illness for Survivors
and Those Who Love and Care for Them*

Greg Pacini
Foreword by Peter D. Weiss, MD

REEDY PRESS
St. Louis, Missouri

Reedy Press
PO Box 5131, St. Louis, MO 63139, USA

For information on Reedy Press publications
visit our website at http://www.reedypress.com.

Library of Congress Cataloging-in-Publication Data: on file

This book is printed on acid-free paper.

ISBN: 0-9753180-6-3

Design by Ellie Jones, MathisJones Communications
Cover Design by Ellie Jones and William Mathis, MathisJones Communications
Photography by Cary Horton
Author Photograph by Bob Morrison
Printed in Canada
05   06   07   08   09   5   4   3   2   1

To the valiant Jean Marie Miller, whose journey
spoke in unique ways to so many individual
hearts and informed millions of the silent
symptoms of ovarian cancer.

Contents

Acknowledgments

Survivors, caregivers, and medical professionals, as students of illness, you have become my greatest teachers. The truth beyond words that you have shared has renovated my soul. Dad and Mom, by continually developing your own spirits, you have fostered the same in me. You are remarkable individuals. Phil, Mary, and Tony, you formed me, and so too my work. PMAC, thanks for your unwavering support of this project.

Thanks to those who graciously studied drafts of this manuscript and provided important feedback: Harold Benjamin, PhD; Clare Boehmer, ASC; Paula Geiss, RN, MSN; Bill Gurley; Lorraine Langdon-Hull, MSW; and Kim Thiboldeaux. Special thanks to Janice Thorup for the conscientious and thorough editing of the first version of this text, and Linda Wendling of Wordbench for the expertise in editing the second version, which took this book to the next level.

Thanks to Josh Stevens, Matt Heidenry, and all those associated with Reedy Press for your talent and for sharing the birth pains of this work. Bob Morrison, you are a kind man and a magician behind the portrait camera. Thank you Cary Horton for the cover photo and images throughout the book, which add richness to the text.

Suzanne Mahon, RN, DNSc, AOCN, APNG, your review of this work gave me important encouragement. Thank you. Don and Kay Young, you have already given so much to those making their way through illness. Thank you for helping here, too.

Dr. David Spiegel, your response had a strong and valuable impact on me. Thanks for your honest and supportive reaction to the material you reviewed.

Dr. Peter Weiss, thank you for your respect and generous spirit. Many benefit from those qualities in you. And thank you for bringing your heart to this book.

Finally, thank you, Joey, for all you are teaching us.

Foreword

Illness touches every one of us in profound ways. We are all destined to experience life-altering, sometimes life-ending illness, or care for loved ones who are facing these same challenges. Medical science, through varied therapeutic modalities, has been able to successfully treat—and even cure—some of these diseases. Despite these advances, we are ill-equipped to adequately support and nurture the psyche through this process. *Journey Beyond Diagnosis* gives us the roadmap, the comforting guide to navigate this treacherous road—for illness survivors, caregivers, and medical professionals.

As a medical oncologist, I have been privileged to lead many patients and their families through the diagnosis, treatment, and outcome of their cancer. During this journey, I particularly emphasize the difficult-to-appreciate "silver lining" of illness—the sudden realization of "what is important," the deepening and strengthening of relationships, and the spiritual awakening—that can act as a support and enable patients to endure the emotional and physical stress of treatment. Throughout, it is the people who offer support—family, friends, physicians, therapists—who are so vital to this healing process.

Through the aid of an allegorical journey, Greg Pacini has provided a means to navigate this very complex emotional, psychological, and physical path. He gives nurturing advice and helpful exercises to get us beyond mere coping—he gives us a map to integrate healing, truth in relationships, and growth as human beings.

This book is an important read, and emotional guide, for all of us—patients, caregivers, medical professionals, therapists—for we all, in some manner, must travel this path. We can all learn and utilize the powerful insights provided in this book.

Peter D. Weiss, MD

Introduction

As you open this book, a recent diagnosis may still have you reeling. You may be in the middle of treatment, and the traveling is tough. Your journey may have thankfully ended with successful surgery. Or you might be seeking a better understanding of the experience of being diagnosed with an illness for professional reasons. Maybe your wife just survived a heart attack. Perhaps your child has been diagnosed with autism. Maybe you or your loved one completed treatment years ago, but the emotional, relational, mental, or spiritual effects on both of you continue. Perhaps you're making this journey alone and want some direction. Or, though your body may not be cured, maybe you have decided to keep traveling. Each of these journeys beyond diagnosis is different. Each has its own meaning and power and pain.

This guide is offered to support you along your way, wherever and however you journey. The pages that follow look closely at the survivor's journey beyond diagnosis. Special chapters and sections for caregivers and medical professionals are provided. Whether a survivor, caregiver, or medical professional, this book is designed to broaden your understanding of each of these points of view, and make your journey better. The Rest Stop chapters benefit all readers, providing step-by-step techniques for managing anxiety, conflict, depression, stress, and emotional fatigue.

Reading sections of this book may be uncomfortable. Survivors, caregivers, and medical professionals all sometimes seek support outside their usual circles because they don't feel safe talking about difficult matters there. This book intentionally moves right into those harder issues. The purpose is to provide a vehicle for going through these roadblocks, rather than around. Often just on the other side of such barriers is the very life sought, which was hidden by the difficulties. In this way, barriers become bridges.

When you've finished reading this book, I hope you'll know better what to expect on the journey beyond diagnosis. Next, I hope you'll have some useable tools for making your journey more comfortable. Finally, I hope you'll sense that you have company for the trip, whether you're a survivor, caregiver, or medical professional.

As a psychotherapist, my work addresses the heart, the mind, and the spirit, in relationship to the body. Case studies presented in this book may make connections between all these parts of the self. However, it is assumed that illness has many sources, including environment and heredity, and that you are not to blame for your illness. Blame has no place in this text.

Finally, it has been said that an illness survivor is anyone who takes a breath after being diagnosed. That is how survivor is defined in this book. You may be two days or twenty years post-diagnosis. And the term survivor is used knowing full well that human beings diagnosed with illness are so much more than their diseases.

Journey
Beyond
Diagnosis

Greg Pacini

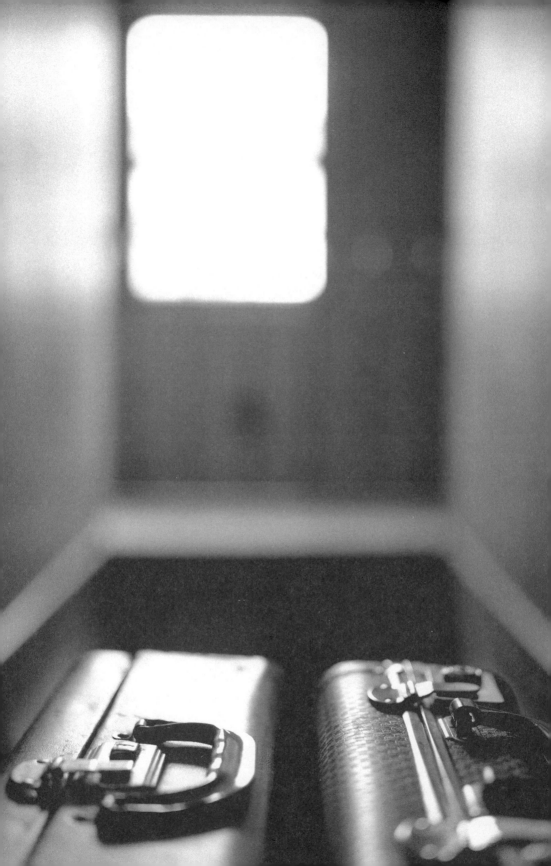

Chapter One

Packing: Preparing for the Journey

*L*ike most trips, the journey beyond diagnosis begins before you actually leave home: things to get ready and things to pack. With some trips, you have plenty of time for that. For other trips, however, there is barely time to throw your clothes in a travel bag. So, let's get started with a look at the issues of readiness and packing.

You may have been readied by your own body and knew you had an illness before hearing the diagnosis. It's not uncommon. Scientifically, you didn't know. But in some other way you did. Maybe there were unusual, minor physical sensations or obvious, powerful symptoms you couldn't miss. Perhaps it was quiet intuition. And then you just knew.

People like you may not be surprised when told, "You have MS"—or cancer, heart disease, or one of so many other diagnosed illnesses. As a matter of fact, folks like you often report feeling relieved: "Now I know I'm not crazy." You have been tracking curious pains, sensations, and gut feelings for a while. You knew.

If you knew before the diagnosis, you may have begun packing then: getting ready emotionally, mentally, relationally, or even spiritually. Perhaps you felt a rush of clarity and strength, deeply aware of what was being called for at this moment in your life. You may have felt a shift in the way you viewed the people you care about. Maybe you started to act differently with them—more loving or more distant. Perhaps you felt terribly alone with the thought of having an illness. Maybe you found a trusted person you could tell about your fear.

You may have rallied your faith in something or some-one, or just sat and wondered. You may have fought wave after wave of feeling, or perhaps you stepped out of that ocean altogether. Maybe you caught yourself spending hours on the Internet. Perhaps you subtly asked many questions, testing a sixth sense against some harder reality.

In preparing, you may have withdrawn from your usual ways, or maybe you noticed yourself racing. Perhaps you began to pack away your hope. Did you box up your fear, confusion, disillusionment, anger, or sadness? Did you pack for your family?

But then again, maybe you were one of those folks who didn't have time to pack. The words of your diagnosis came as a complete surprise. All of a sudden you were on a journey. Nobody told you that you were going, but things were beginning to move, and move quickly. Did you wonder who was driving? Did you hope it wasn't you?

Was there a sense of sureness about the journey, or did you wish you had a map?

At the start, there were doctors to see, tests to sched-ule, and procedures to be run. You had to establish treat-ment protocols, and then get going with that. Consequently, *you may have packed the initial wave of feel-ings*, knowing you needed strength to contend with all the external activity.

And what about the *internal* activity? What about bouts of sadness and terror, and so much more? Well, when first diagnosed, a lot of people move with instinct. Like trying to catch a ball that they're not ready for— reacting and hoping to handle it. After this initial reflex, some say to themselves, "I can do this, I've handled worse." Others collapse quietly alone somewhere. Some cry. Some die inside for a minute. Some, way down in there someplace, whisper, "Why me?" Others proclaim, "Why not me!?" Many seek comfort in an explanation. Many pray. Some push others out of the way and say, "Let me do the driving." Still others make absolutely certain that their circle of support is tight and close.

Some stuff all the courage, trust, love, confidence, and peace they can possibly fit in their emotional suitcase. Others pack shame: "I brought this on with my own hectic life," or, ". . . my cigarettes"; "They say stress causes cancer. I did this to myself." Others pack blame: "My kids are outta control. If it wasn't for all the pressure they cause me. . . ." Or, "I inherited this. It's not my fault." Many pack some trust *and* some fear.

These are all possible thoughts, feelings, and responses to the start of the journey beyond diagnosis. Each has its place. There are others. But in the beginning, it's more about action and less about thinking or feeling. So you pack. It's OK. Packing is an example of *emotional efficiency*. We'll discuss this more later.

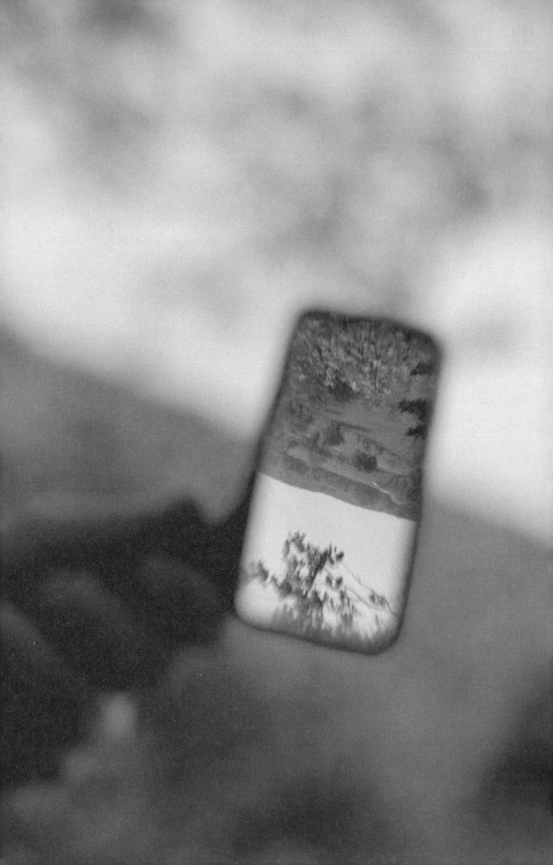

Chapter Two

Leaving Home: The Familiar

Once you're ready and packed, you leave home. And what is home? Home is where you dangle your legs off the kitchen counter late at night, eatin' a cold piece of chicken while your spouse has homemade coffee cake. When things are good, home is a place of comfort, peace, passion, acceptance, and familiarity. Home is a place you know.

When diagnosed with illness, you leave home—you leave the familiar. You leave the comfort of a well-known way of life for a place about which you know little. When you leave this metaphorical home, this place of comfort, what else is left behind?

Some leave behind a fear they lived with all their lives. From some seemingly unknown place, a strength surfaces beyond compare. Other illness survivors, especially when first diagnosed, leave their peace and hope.

Some leave the rocky road of troubled relationships. Almost like magic, the diagnosis has lifted years of marital problems or tension within a family, as all unite to take on the illness. Others leave relationships outright, trusting such decisions might make them feel better, and better able to take on the illness.

Then there are those travelers who stay in relationships but leave some of the connectedness they felt there. Karen was twenty-seven when she heard the words, "Your white cell counts are very elevated. Further testing is needed, but it's most likely you have leukemia. I'm sorry." It was only three or four sessions into our work together when Karen reported a change in how she was acting with her two daughters.

"I'm finding things to do on the weekends so I don't have to be at home with the girls," Karen shared.

"How do you understand this change?" I asked.

"I think it helps me to just stay busy, but I'm not sure. The whole things scares me," Karen blurted.

"Consider gently listening to what's going on inside you the next few times you make plans that don't include your girls. Those feelings may have something to tell you," I suggested.

It wasn't long before Karen began to unpeel her emotions about the changing relationship with her daughters. Yes, staying busy did help her. Then she realized that there was a pain under the busyness. The pain was strongest around her girls. Eventually, she discovered a collision between her love for her daughters and the fear of something happening to herself. She was unconsciously leaving her children a little bit at a time, to lessen the blow of a permanent separation she feared.

In time, Karen also uncovered a feeling—at an even deeper level—that really surprised her. She felt a tinge of jealousy for the exuberance and carefree ways of people that she saw in public places like malls and schoolyards. She even admitted some of this same jealousy for her life-loving daughters. Driven by all these feelings, Karen had left home: *left the more familiar*, connected relationship she had with her children before the diagnosis.

Other survivors leave a trust felt for their own bodies—the solid ground of believing the body will tell them when something is really amiss. Most don't realize they walked around in this trust. Some pull away from their God. Some say goodbye to their sense of invincibility.

Many depart from a feeling of control about life. Others move away from believing they're a part of the "normal world." Some step away from their joy, their playfulness. For many, independence and self-assurance seem like they've been left behind.

Finally, some disconnect from a mind that can sometimes be still, concentrate, or remember. They disconnect from a deep knowing that A plus B does equal C. And those closest to the person diagnosed typically detach from many of the very same things—sometimes more.

❖ ❖ ❖

It is important to remember that the trip is just beginning. Leaving something behind doesn't mean you can't return to it later. However, by talking about what is left behind, there is an acknowledgment of what may be true at this moment. Acknowledgment, in and of itself, can be healing.

"Leaving things behind" at this point in the journey is really the experience of loss, and loss brings its own set of feelings. But with so much external activity at the start of the journey beyond diagnosis, this loss—this internal activity that is equally complex—often goes unnoticed. This is a first-things-first scenario. It's as if the *whole person* carries wisdom for these times, recognizing that the volume of thoughts and feelings present with a diagnosis could easily overwhelm. And the wisdom also knows that if the body is not tended to first, foremost, and with full available energy, then the body might suffer severe consequences. So, at the beginning of the journey beyond diagnosis, like most trips, the focus is on packing and then on leaving home.

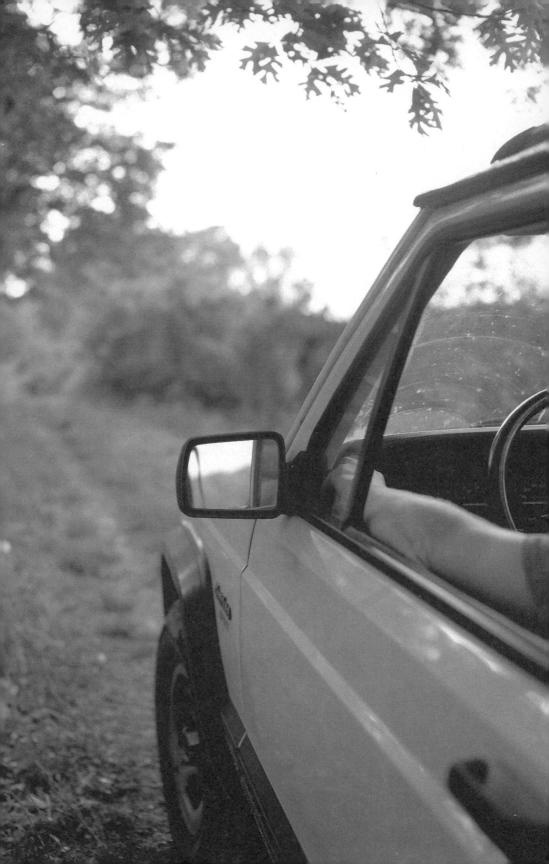

Chapter Three

On the Road: Beginning the Treatment Process

*N*ow that the bags have been packed and loaded, and you've left home, "movement" begins by responding medically to the illness. What is there to be done once on this road of the journey beyond diagnosis?

Finding the Right Doctor

The travels often start with finding the right doctor. Many seek the doctor with the best set of skills. Some search the Internet or network with friends hoping to find, for example, the surgeon with the best track record for the procedure they need. Others want a doctor with not only good technical skills but also with good bedside manner. To them, this is as important as technical talent. Interestingly enough, articles like the one found in the journal, *Medical Care,* suggest that the nature of the relationship between patient and doctor may impact physical outcomes.[1] These articles support the notion that *the relationships* with physicians or medical teams may themselves be healing. Relationship is a powerful factor in health, and that includes relationship with medical professionals during the journey beyond diagnosis.

Jeff was a fifty-nine-year-old nurse recently diagnosed with hepatitis C, contracted from a needle stick at work. He began counseling with me about ten months after his diagnosis—certainly "on the road." Jeff had been professionally taking care of people all his adult life.

When immersed in the experience of being "taken care of" himself by a medical team, Jeff realized something about his own behavior.

Working past his uncomfortable emotion, Jeff revealed, "I wouldn't wish this disease on anybody. But it's changed me."

"How so?" I asked.

"I've spent all my life caring for others. When this disease forced me to surrender to care *from* others, I felt this sort of melting in me. I didn't understand it at first. Actually, I resisted it," Jeff said.

"You resisted what?" was my next question.

"I resisted," Jeff continued, "letting myself get taken care of by this medical team. It's not something I've really ever had a lot of. But here's the thing. Once I let go to their care, it was like medicine to me. That's when I realized this was what I was looking for in all my years of giving to others."

"Help me with that," I replied.

With strength, Jeff finished, "In caring for others all these years, I've been giving what I've always wanted to get."

For Jeff, healing came from not only the medicine but from those who gave it to him. The relationship between Jeff and his medical team, from that point forward, impacted how he operated in the world. This can happen on the recovery road.

The Treatment Plan

Jeff's physical recovery included the treatment plan—another aspect of being on the road of the journey beyond diagnosis. Depending on the illness, treatment plans may involve surgery, a protracted medication regimen, or both. You may require physical therapies, occupational therapies, chemotherapies, or radiation therapies. There might be treatments done beforehand to make surgery possible.

Some survivors choose conventional medical practices, while others explore only alternative methods, and still others combine modalities.

And once the actual therapies and procedures have been elected, specific *protocols within the treatment plan must be established.* This may involve selecting which particular drugs or combination of drugs will be used, or if radiation is involved, which parts of the body will be treated. Questions are answered about frequency and duration of each treatment, the number of treatment cycles, and the amount of time between cycles.

Starting treatment is usually a significant step down the road beyond diagnosis. Beginning the treatment process usually includes multiple office or hospital visits, follow-up tests, treatment changes, and ways to alleviate side effects. And, as Chapter 5 explores, all this may come packed with an emotional component.

Asking Questions of the Medical Team

Asking questions of the medical team is an important part of the road traveled beyond diagnosis for many, and it may continue well past treatment. While some resist asking questions, medical professionals often find guidance for a patient's treatment through that patient or caregiver's questions. More importantly, questions answered often means reduced stress, and this may actually support the survivor's physical recovery.

Many survivors bring a caregiver to appointments to listen with the objectivity that the survivor sometimes can't muster. Survivors then allow the caregiver to ask questions for them. Or survivors might simply have the caregiver back them up on topics or issues they, in the anxiety often present during doctor visits, might overlook. Some survivors and caregivers bring lists of questions to appointments to be sure all the vital uncertainties are cleared. The simple act of self-respect shown by seeking answers to questions most important to you can improve morale. Questions show up about unidentified pain, curious side effects, and length of treatment, among others.

Questions common when a little farther down the road include, "Who's the best person to talk with on the treatment team when I want answers?" and, "How do I plan my life around this treatment?"

Changes in Relationships

If relationships are an important part of well-being and an important part of the recovery road, then changes in relationships surely are as well. In the early goings, these changes may take on uncommon appearances. Eric's forty-year-old daughter was diagnosed with lupus fourteen months earlier.

"Some part of me thinks she should just get on with her life. And yet I know she's scared," Eric expressed. "I don't really know what's best for her. Should I push her or hold her?"

These are the questions of people trying to find their place for the journey, not unlike the shifting and turning that families do in the early part of a long drive. Relationships are shifting and turning. Everyone is figuring out how to relate to the illness survivor and each other: "Will I call a lot or just send cards?"; "Will I ask about the illness or just talk about everyday things?"

When you literally travel on a long drive, everyone is usually wide awake for the first hundred miles. There's a kind of united focus, whether or not it's discussed. All are intent on the journey itself. There's chatter in the car about where you're going and how you're going to get there. Nonetheless, most of the attention is on the here and now, and what's to come.

The same is true with the journey beyond diagnosis. The news of an illness usually draws people together with a common goal and united focus. What is typically talked about in the beginning is the here and now, where you're headed and how you're going to get there. That is, doing everything possible, in the best way possible, to treat or get rid of the illness. This is all part of the *external activity*—part of getting down the road.

Chapter 5 will begin to take a closer look at all that may be going on *inside* you as you move down the road on the journey beyond diagnosis—the *internal activity*. But before undertaking that leg of the journey, a nice beverage or snack may be in order.

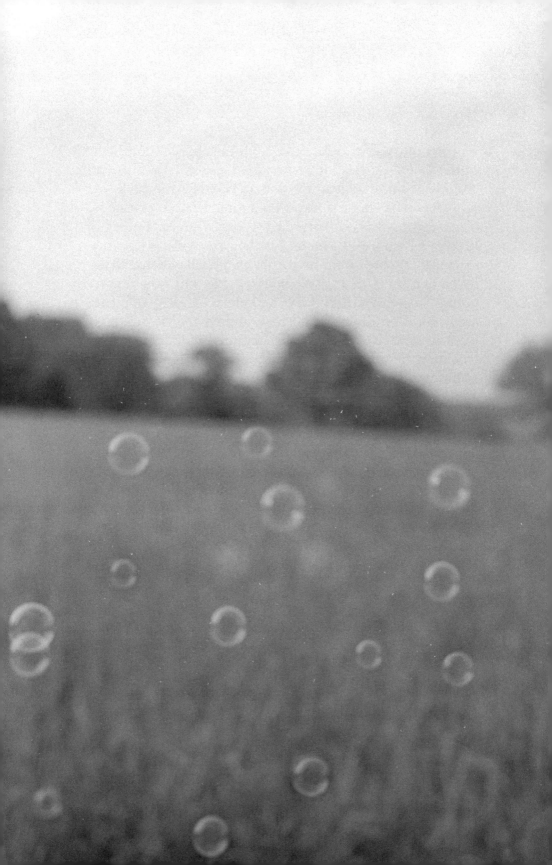

Chapter Four

Refreshments: Little Ways to Take Care of Yourself

Are you one of those folks on road trips that digs into the chocolates or those organic blue corn tortillas chips before you leave the driveway? With the journey beyond diagnosis, it's a good idea to hit the refreshments of heart early and often. Snacking on the kind of refreshments that we're talking about in this chapter helps refresh the spirit and maintain focus. It's an understatement to say that the journey beyond an illness diagnosis can drain you. Without attention to those things that *return* energy, strength, focus, and motivation, travelers may find it difficult to finish the trip.

So here's an opportunity, by reading the list of "snacks" below, to check your cooler and see how you're doing when it comes to maintaining your strength—a few refreshments, if you please:

❖ Study the stars
❖ Tickle a child
❖ Cut the grass
❖ Listen to laughter
❖ Paint
❖ Pray
❖ Walk to the mailbox
❖ Make cookies
❖ Write a letter
❖ Go to work
❖ Leave work
❖ Study the faces of those you love
❖ Volunteer

- ❖ Just sit
- ❖ Work on your car
- ❖ Knit
- ❖ Play catch
- ❖ Play poker
- ❖ Read
- ❖ Go to your counselor
- ❖ Talk with your nurse
- ❖ Talk with another survivor
- ❖ Sing in the wind
- ❖ Burn sage
- ❖ Practice your violin
- ❖ Dance in the snow
- ❖ Fiddle
- ❖ Dance in the arms of someone you love
- ❖ Work a crossword puzzle
- ❖ Pat your dog on the head
- ❖ Kiss your baby's cheek
- ❖ Crank up the music
- ❖ Hold your lover closer than you ever have
- ❖ Lay in the sun
- ❖ Call your grandfather
- ❖ Look through old pictures
- ❖ Take new ones
- ❖ Look soulfully at your life
- ❖ Share your thoughts with someone you trust
- ❖ Break sticks and yell
- ❖ Go to a farm and talk to the horses
- ❖ Hit the gym
- ❖ Have a beer
- ❖ Write a letter to someone you respect, with your weaker hand
- ❖ Cut out all the pictures you can find that remind you of you
- ❖ Give them to your mate

- ❖ Drum
- ❖ Sit on the floor and have a sandwich with your child
- ❖ Notice how your hands work
- ❖ Turn off your telephone
- ❖ Close your e-mail account
- ❖ Open one
- ❖ Ask someone to help you
- ❖ Help someone
- ❖ Fly in your mind
- ❖ Stand with your feet in the sand
- ❖ Collect rocks that mean something to you
- ❖ Lie flat on your back but not in your bed
- ❖ Color
- ❖ Throw darts
- ❖ Throw a football
- ❖ Throw a party tomorrow
- ❖ Throw out the junk in your house
- ❖ Throw your arms around somebody
- ❖ Throw a fit
- ❖ Throw your cares to the wind and see where they land
- ❖ Live for a day like you were somebody else
- ❖ Learn from it
- ❖ Teach somebody what you learned
- ❖ Learn to love something new
- ❖ Make up a song and sing it in the shower
- ❖ Shower with your clothes on
- ❖ Invite your spouse to come in and take them off
- ❖ Turn the lights off and watch the darkness
- ❖ Talk to the darkness
- ❖ Speak of the light
- ❖ Listen
- ❖ Love every part of yourself
- ❖ Tell the truth

- ❖ Own what you don't particularly care for about you
- ❖ Confess
- ❖ Believe in something important
- ❖ Write about those beliefs
- ❖ Write a book
- ❖ Date your wife
- ❖ Dazzle somebody
- ❖ Do it without words
- ❖ Wait at the door for something wonderful to arrive and pretend it gets there
- ❖ Deliver an important message to the world driving home
- ❖ Clap your hands for the hell of it
- ❖ Take a bow while you're there
- ❖ Ride a train
- ❖ Ride off into the sunset for somebody
- ❖ Make your fingers tap
- ❖ Tape a note on your own back that tells people what you need today
- ❖ Smell something new
- ❖ Feed the birds
- ❖ Burn a candle as a gesture of respect
- ❖ Take back your power
- ❖ Gather up something wonderful in your arms
- ❖ Donate
- ❖ Take some time for trimming your nails
- ❖ Be on time
- ❖ Be late
- ❖ Be proud of who you are
- ❖ Be silly
- ❖ Be bold
- ❖ Be wrong
- ❖ Be right
- ❖ Be alone
- ❖ Be surrounded by people who love you

- ❖ Be yourself again
- ❖ Be afraid of nothing for seven minutes
- ❖ Be that person you used to be if only in your mind
- ❖ Be very appreciative of who you've become
- ❖ Be kind
- ❖ Be right back
- ❖ Belong to something
- ❖ Be careful
- ❖ Be carefree
- ❖ Be the apple of someone's eye and ask them to be the same for you
- ❖ Be that ten-year-old boy
- ❖ Pay for someone's dinner without them knowing who
- ❖ Bring home flowers even if you're the only one there
- ❖ Hold your breath and listen to your own heart beat
- ❖ Hold your purse on the other arm
- ❖ Hold hands for a long, long time
- ❖ Hold back, let it go
- ❖ Hold something very precious for just a second
- ❖ Hold a meeting and let everybody know how you want to do this, whatever this is
- ❖ Have a piece of fruit, only make each bite last fifteen seconds
- ❖ Do some chocolate
- ❖ While we're on food, bake a cake for the first time
- ❖ Carry a piece of chopped wood
- ❖ Take a nap
- ❖ Take another nap
- ❖ Tell somebody you did
- ❖ Have them join you
- ❖ Make a mountain out of a mole hill for fun
- ❖ Spell everything backwards
- ❖ Box with your boyfriend

- ❖ Be gentle
- ❖ Be vital if only for that long
- ❖ Give it a try
- ❖ Try it again tomorrow
- ❖ Make a paper airplane
- ❖ Forgive yourself for good
- ❖ Fix a little something
- ❖ Fast if your doctor thinks it's OK
- ❖ If not, just give something up
- ❖ Celebrate being sober
- ❖ Be more powerful than you ever have
- ❖ Tear up
- ❖ Touch someone's lips with your own
- ❖ Watch a stupid movie
- ❖ Take five every time you can
- ❖ Work hard and feel the rich joy
- ❖ Pat somebody on the back in a way that really touches them, you know, mean it
- ❖ Be kind with it
- ❖ Think about the moon
- ❖ Forgive anybody you want
- ❖ Cover your plants when it gets cold
- ❖ Let your children know you can be strong and loving
- ❖ Carry it out
- ❖ Tackle something
- ❖ Wave
- ❖ Have a banana split
- ❖ Have a cow
- ❖ Don't stop noticing
- ❖ Count your blessings as contrived as that might seem
- ❖ Rub some brown, crackly leaves in your hands
- ❖ Let your palms just barely touch the tips of new grass blades

❖ Hear your lover's voice, not the words
❖ Cuddle
❖ Splash in a puddle
❖ Find someplace to watch deer
❖ Tiptoe, trying not to wake
❖ Feel your heart—the emotional part—when saying goodbye to someone
❖ Goof around
❖ Remember who you are
❖ Experience the power of absolute honesty all the time

Anything jump out at you when you read that list? It might be worth paying attention to. It might be worth reading again in a week, to see if your reaction shifts. The shift might be worth paying attention to.

If you're up for more than a snack, take a minute to consider these questions: "How do you care for yourself when you feel stressed?" "What do you do when you're not stressed to prevent becoming stressed?" "What do you do that ignites your spirit?" "What makes you feel loved?" "What makes you feel loving?" "What brings you much gratitude?" "Where, when, and how do you find your peace?" "When you need comfort, how do you get it?" "Who are the people you feel best around?"

If you're still hungry, a later Rest Stop chapter will give you more to chew on. It offers you an exercise with questions like these to measure how well you refresh yourself. But first, now that you've snacked a bit, let's take a closer look at the *internal activity* that often comes with an illness diagnosis.

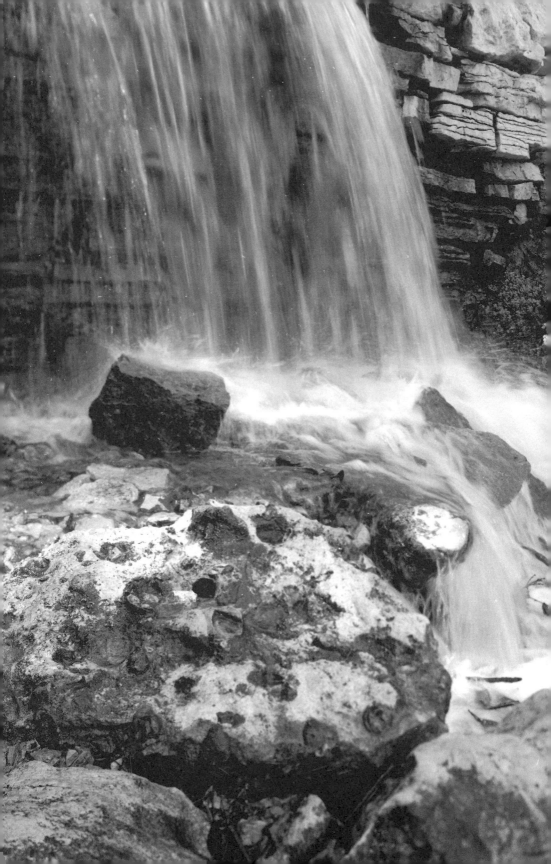

Chapter Five

Improving the Ride: Thoughts About Tough Feelings

Hopefully you feel a bit nourished now. Let's take a look at the *internal activity* or emotions that may accompany the journey beyond diagnosis. Everyone's journey is different. And there's no right or wrong way to travel. This chapter does, however, offer some travel tips.

During the journey beyond diagnosis, there may be times of intense relief and joy, times of utter loss and confusion, times of profound faith and strength, or times of despair and disbelief. Some emotions may be more poignant than others, some more pervasive, others more enduring. But in the beginning of the trip, many feelings get "packed away" inside you, especially if they are difficult. Not unreasonable at the start of the trip. Yet, it also stands to reason that there is only so much the suitcase of your emotional self can hold. We focus here on responding to emotions and the possible connections between emotional health and physical health.

An article in *Social Science and Medicine* tells us that chronic physical conditions affect depression directly, as well as indirectly, by aggravating domestic, occupational, and economic strains, and by undermining personal resources like self-esteem and mastery. [2]

So, illness can take an emotional toll. Consequently, you might want to learn sooner rather than later some ways to keep your emotional luggage from busting open, whether you are a survivor, caregiver, or medical professional.

As a culture, we do well with the "positive" emotions like courage, happiness, and hope. But when it comes to the more difficult feelings like sadness, fear, discouragement, and anger, there's not much of a road map. The model for responding to tough emotions is generally fairly simple. You have your outbursts, your withdrawals, your tears, and your complete shutdowns. These all have their place and price. However, the ride can be very rough when journeying on only these emotional extremes. What's suggested here are new shocks.

A broader range of feelings during the illness journey—or any time for that matter—is like getting better shocks on your car. The ride is smoother because you're not bouncing between emotional extremes. Nor are you locked in a stiff set of fairly flat reactions. With better emotional shock absorbers, the road hasn't changed, but the vehicle of your emotional self has.

Historically, tough feelings like sadness, fear, and disappointment have been described as "negative." And yet, it's very possible to think of *all* emotions as positive since each acts as a signpost pointing to what works for you, and what doesn't. In other words, all emotions teach.

It is only natural to have difficult emotions when dealing with diagnosed illness. Giving yourself permission to honor these feelings as they occur is part of an *authentic* journey. Unfortunately, having an *authentic* recovery experience has become confused with having a *bad attitude*. Consequently, many survivors find themselves contending with more than their illness. They may find themselves also wrestling with the people who insist they "just stay positive." As a result, survivors can wind up grappling with the uncertainty that these well-intended demands create, not to mention grappling with the emotions themselves. Of course, those doing the insisting are usually trying to be loving.

Boy, this all gets so confusing. The word on the street is, "Attitude is everything. Stay positive." The fact is, when on the journey beyond diagnosis, positive is not always what you feel. Tough feelings do surface and, as we will discuss later in the chapter, just making room for the harder feelings may have a positive impact on your physical self. Here's a story describing some of the layers of difficult emotions that can show up with an illness experience.

Audrey had been surviving surgery from a leg sarcoma for about eight months when she began attending counseling. It was now a year after that first session. Before her diagnosis, Audrey was very active with full-time employment and a family. She enjoyed hiking and runs through the woods with her dog. The illness had taken her right leg, from just below the knee.

Early psychotherapy focused on Audrey's anger and sadness. These feelings came in alternating waves. Then she began to grieve. She mourned the loss of her limb first. Then Audrey grieved all the less obvious losses that often come with losing some part of the body: loss of physical freedom, loss of body image, loss of independence, loss of dreams, loss of esteem, loss of favorite activities and clothes, and more. Audrey even lost a familiar gate, stance, and posture.

With time, however, Audrey eventually recovered much of the self she felt disconnected from early on. Getting comfortable with a prosthetic leg made a big difference. The sadness and anger began to lift. As her mourning turned to living, and Audrey felt times of real joy again, another set of emotions surfaced that seemed somehow vaguely familiar.

"I've spent thirty-eight years running around, hopping from one thing to the next," Audrey revealed. "God, I can never stand still. And I get it now. It scares me to death to stand still. If I stand still, I might notice how sad I am," she said.

So Audrey and I explored early life experiences that represented another kind of loss that she had never really mourned. It is frequently true that beneath emotions occurring naturally with an illness, there are related emotions that are much older. At times like these, the emotional "suitcase" may feel like it's going to bust. "Unpacking" some of these feelings may help. The next chapter offers an exercise showing you how to respond to emotions in general. Later chapters offer techniques for managing specific emotions like anxiety and depression. Before reading and practicing these exercises, you might find some additional information about emotional and physical health useful.

It was my good fortune to hear David Spiegel, MD, a professor at Stanford University, speak at a luncheon for an organization that serves illness survivors. Spiegel's work with metastatic cancer survivors was featured on Bill Moyers's PBS series, *Healing and the Mind*. His luncheon message was clear: Always being positive is a misguided response when confronted with illness.

But this message may leave you, as a survivor, caregiver, or medical professional, with some pointed questions: "Am I going to hurt myself by feeling sad or angry or disappointed or confused?" "Will allowing this broader range of emotions, as suggested in this book, work against me?"

Rollin McCraty, director of research for the Institute

for Heartmath, states in a *Natural Health* article, "People who maintain an inner feeling of anger in the form of a slow burn actually extend the suppression of their immune system." He reports that outbursts also negatively impact immune function.[3] They key seems to be balance.

Furthermore, a 2001 article in *Neuroendocrinology Letters* indicates that stress, anxiety, and depressive states are associated with a weakening of the immune system, and with the enhanced frequency of tumors.[4] Of course, in reading this most people may think, "Well, then I can't allow myself to be stressed, anxious, or depressed." And yet, as the next chapter points out, stress, anxiety, and depression all seem to persist when you continuously attempt to push them away. The research is suggesting that this pushing away or holding down of difficult emotions is hard on your body. This pushing away is essentially the same thing as "packing." Again, balance is the best bet. Good emotional "shocks" provide that.

What's recommended here is that you sometimes go through rather than around painful emotions. This is not to say that you should replace conventional treatment with an emotional journey to cure your illness. Whatever means you employ to heal your body, *you are on* an emotional journey. One does not eliminate the need for the other.

There is no question that the way you manage the emotional part of your journey beyond diagnosis *will* affect the quality of your life. So, why not manage those emotions in a way that *improves* that quality? As a bonus, science is telling us that well-handled emotions may support whatever treatments you are pursuing to heal your disease. And well-handled emotions always support healing of your spirit.

The process of going through difficult emotions could be thought of as a *different* way of being positive. *Going through* difficult feelings sooner rather than later can sometimes mitigate depression and anxiety and prevent the buildup that leads to responding in extreme emotional ways, like outbursts, withdrawal, ongoing tears, or complete emotional shut downs.

This *going-through* process may do more than improve your emotional ride. It can, in a sense, unclog an emotional section of the self's fuel line. You then may find you have the energy needed to move forward. That can feel pretty positive. That's what allowing the "negative" feelings to move through you can do.

Having said all that, science also tells us a "good attitude" does matter. This is part of why the whole "be positive" notion gets so confusing. Like most of life, it is never simply one way or the other. In addition to successful medical treatment, effective recovery seems to include *both* authenticity (i.e., letting yourself experience some of the tough feelings as they pass through you) and some form of "being positive." Goal setting, forward thinking, and seeing yourself well can make a difference in your morale and your body.

For example, a 2002 study cited in *Stress: The International Journal on the Biology of Stress* reports that patients who received six weeks of training in visualization, (seeing themselves well) "up-regulated" or strengthened their immune systems, most notably the increased production of natural killer cells, which play a vital role in fighting illness.[5] The visualizations worked.

Additionally, a 2003 article in *Seminars in Clinical*

Neuropsychiatry reports that hypnotic-like methods involving relaxation, suggestion, and imagery have significant impact on cancer-related pain.[6] Attitude and mind can influence the body.

Bottom line, as tough feelings surface during your journey beyond diagnosis—and they are going to surface—let them move through you. Try not to get stuck in any feeling, but give each its due. Emotions are important signposts, but not the destination. Churchill said, "If you're going through hell, keep going." Visit the emotional pain, but don't pitch a tent there. Trust yourself. And allow and encourage the hope, joy, strength, and wellness you seek.

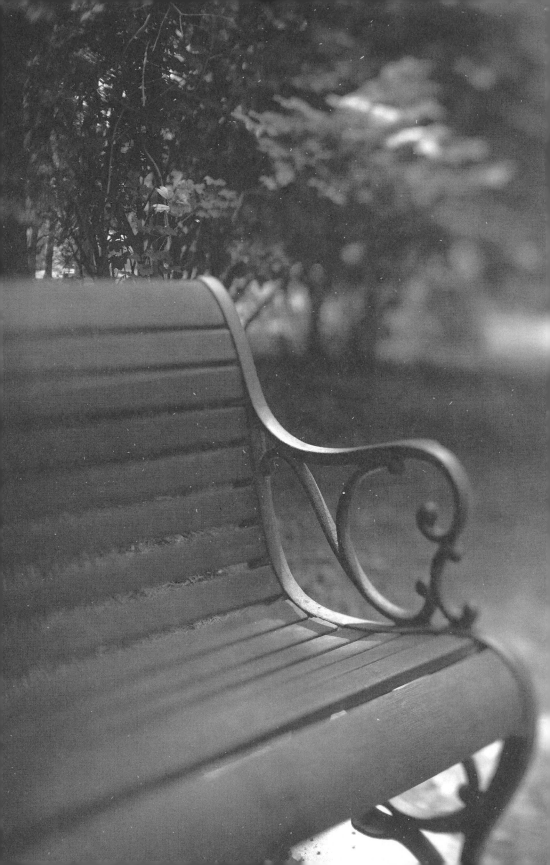

Chapter Six

Rest Stop #1: Triple A–The Simple Tool for Responding to Tough Feelings

*L*ike any long drive, there are always places along the way to take a break. You can either pull off and rest or keep going. The same is true with the journey beyond diagnosis. This chapter, like other Rest Stop chapters, is designed to help you rest. It offers information and a step-by-step technique that might make you and your life more comfortable.

In the previous chapter, better shock absorbers were discussed—greater emotional range. One way to establish greater emotional range is to emotionally "unpack." In the interest of smoothing out your ride, I'd like to introduce you to ways to befriend your tough feelings. That is, unpack some of them.

"Whoa! No thanks. I don't need friends like that," you're thinking. OK. That's fair. But when unequipped to work through all the tough feelings that can show up with a diagnosis, your range of emotion is limited. With limited emotional range, you're like a car with poor shocks. A little bump and you're bottoming out. Or, so stiff that steering through difficult curves is dangerous. Either way, there's less stability.

This chapter explores ways to befriend difficult feelings in general. Later chapters will address ways to respond to specific, tough feelings like anxiety, depression, and anger. Here is a three-step technique—Triple A—to help you "unpack" some of the difficult emotions you may be carrying on your journey beyond diagnosis.

Triple A

Step 1. Acknowledge
Step 2. Accept
Step 3. Act

Step 1. Acknowledge

Until feelings of sadness, anger, frustration, or confusion are acknowledged, nothing changes. The uncomfortableness persists. Uncomfortable and persistent feelings that are not identified may go underground. Therese Rando calls this kind of emotional response *avoidance.*[7]

Avoidance seems like a very negative word. And yet, at times there can be wisdom in avoiding significant, difficult feelings, especially early on. For example, it is often emotionally _inefficient_ for people to dive head first into the turbulence of their emotions in the beginning, when lots of external tasks need to be accomplished. Only so much can be managed at once. At times like these, it may be emotionally *efficient* to keep the emotions hidden. People will more likely treat you just like they always have, so you can get through, for example, an event at your child's school.

Trouble may brew, however, if the tough feelings along the journey are never considered. When feelings go underground, they can manage you rather than you managing them. More often than not, hidden, difficult feelings express themselves through behavior. You may buzz around, trying to stay on the surface of your life, or you may find yourself lethargic because precious energy is spent working to keep unexpressed feelings below the surface.

Other survivors, caregivers, and even medical professionals may have angry outbursts as the hidden levels of feelings build up and release. Some eventually withdraw from others, or shut down the emotional self all together.

So the first step in preventing the buildup that can lead to emotional bottoming out is to **acknowledge** what is going on inside you: acknowledge that something is out of sync.

To acknowledge that you feel some difficult things somewhere inside is no more than what it is. This step is not about doing anything with those feelings. It is only about noticing them. The process of noticing is perhaps the simplest but most profound and effective of all the therapeutic tools. Noticing feelings is like having a wise and gentle observer inside. This observer brings no judgment or pressure to change what is noticed. The observer does nothing more than see what is there. That's all!

Step 2. Accept

When people learn to acknowledge what is really happening inside, sometimes frustration, disappointment, or shame for what they find follows: "I can't believe I'm still letting this get to me." That's why this step makes a difference. If you don't accept all that you uncover inside, a battle may ensue between who you are and who you think you should be. This Triple A exercise, and this book for that matter, has nothing to do with *shoulds, coulds, or ought to be's.* By simply embracing whatever you find inside your emotional self, the process of "going through" can continue.

But this kind of unconditionality for self can feel foreign and unusual. So much of our world insists that when something is awry, it must be changed. With this mindset, the idea of *just accepting* all that you find inside may feel like you're not doing enough—like things aren't going to improve. It might even feel like accepting feelings is giving them more power. On the contrary, by acknowledging and accepting all that you feel, those difficult emotions are often disempowered, and as we discussed in the last chapter, that might help your immune system. Acknowledging and accepting tough feelings is an antidote to suppressing them.

It's a little like putting a dog in your basement—not a particularly friendly dog, but not a mean dog either. If you forget that the dog's down there, beware. After a while, when you do go back, there's gonna be a mess. Wait even longer, and the dog could turn on you. But if you befriend the dog, it won't get mean. The dog might even support you. Attending to tough feelings may help prevent them from making a mess inside you or worse, doing some emotional damage. Giving your feelings attention can improve the quality of your life.

Here is another benefit from simply acknowledging and accepting your feelings. When you witness and accept feelings, you become an observer of yourself. Consequently, *you* are no longer sad or fearful or hopeless. Only *a part of you* is. Essentially, you enter the eye of the storm. In this way it is possible to be quiet within yourself, even in the presence of strong emotions. From this quiet place, choice becomes possible, and that changes everything. Yet when you are simply caught up in emotion, without the "witness" self, there is only reaction, and choice is out of the picture.

So, by not really doing anything with your feelings beyond *acknowledging* them and *accepting* them, you really are doing something. But when you consistently circle around your tough feelings by ignoring them, those feelings stack up, creating a wall between you and a life of genuine joy, strength, courage, and hope. Acknowledging and accepting the bricks of your difficult emotions removes the wall, giving you access to a more comfortable life waiting inside.

Consider for a second what **accepting** a feeling might sound like? If your internal and objective observer could speak, it might have this to share about your sadness: "I am sad right now. I could start crying. I know it's because I can't see my grandkids today, with my counts so low. I accept this sadness in the moment." When you look directly at your feelings like this, they move on more quickly.

The neutral and internal witness might say this about your fear: "I haven't had a blood test in two months. I'm about to jump out of my skin, I'm so anxious about what's happening inside me. Yes, it is hard to trust my body right now."

Finally, inner acceptance of anger might go like this: "I would give anything to walk across the room right now. I am so angry that I can't do anything more than just sit here. I have reason to be angry." Now, some of you, as you read this, may be thinking, "Well, that's helpful. It's nothing more than feeling sorry for yourself. You can't just lay around thinking this kind of stuff all day." Guess what. You're right. Well, partly. The truth is, you can sit around and think that kind of stuff all day, if you want. It is a choice. But staying lost in any one difficult feeling may be costly.

However, the point of this whole chapter is that when you simply give yourself permission to notice and embrace the tough feelings, they tend to dissipate. After that, you are less likely to lay around—metaphorically and literally. It is when tough feelings don't get acknowledged that they interfere with your day-to-day life. Unacknowledged, difficult emotions can chew at you from the inside, and this is when people often find themselves listless and unmotivated. Acknowledged and accepted, these feelings pass through, and you're more ready to move.

Step 3. Act

As you begin to experience the power of this "going through" process by *acknowledging* and *accepting* all that you feel, you do start to move and *naturally* do things differently. With feelings cleared, life looks different. With this improved view, you more comfortably respond in new and effective ways. Here's an example of how this change process might unfold when addressing some illness-related emotions.

Say you were diagnosed with non-Hodgkin's lymphoma nine months ago. You have been given some really good news about the illness and you're having moments when your life feels normal. But something isn't right. When you look around outside yourself, you see many people offering genuine support. Your wife is among them. And yet, when you look around inside yourself, you begin to acknowledge that, in addition to feeling thankful and happy for your returning health, some part of you is experiencing a less comfortable emotion. What you feel, and why, is unclear, but by acknowledging the uncomfortableness, something happens. Your senses sharpen about this particular uncomfortableness.

With this keener awareness, you realize that the uncomfortableness is most pointed near the end of the day. Even though you don't like the feeling, you are now accepting it, and it is guiding you. You explore what might be different about the end of the day. Hmmm, the phone doesn't ring as much, the kids are in bed and you and your wife have time alone. Then the understanding gets even clearer. When you go to bed early, you don't feel so uncomfortable. But when you stay up a while with your wife and watch TV, your uncomfortableness builds. So now you recognize that when you are alone with your wife, you feel the most uncomfortable. But that seems odd, because you love her a lot. So you continue to pay attention to your inner life and this odd uncomfortableness.

As you have passing moments with your wife, you notice that sometimes the uncomfortableness that builds at the end of the day appears as flashes throughout the day. One morning, your wife walks past you while you're eating breakfast and says, "When's your next check-up, honey? It's so hard not knowing what's going on with your lymphoma between these doctor visits." You are now very conscious of just how uncomfortable her comment makes you. Then the dominos begin to tumble.

You remember many similar comments your wife made early on. You thought her comments were supporting you. So often they were, especially in the beginning. But now you see her comments as laden with her fear, and you have been growing increasingly uncomfortable with that because your prognosis is very positive. Your uncomfortableness with her fear has gotten so significant that you find it difficult to sit alone with her in the evenings.

Having acknowledged and accepted your own uncomfortableness, new awareness surfaces. Right **action** now seems obvious. So you sit with your wife, whom you love and miss, and share from your heart how you may be pulling away because of the fear she expresses. Yes, there is some uncomfortableness even in the conversation, but she wants to hear you. Eventually, she agrees to work on communicating with less fear. *She becomes aware* that she is still really scared about your illness and decides to speak to your minister about it. She is entitled to be afraid. Before long, the fear and uncomfortableness in your relationship lessens and is eventually replaced with more contact and enjoyment. Your life feels better. So does your wife's.

But if you had not first walked through and cleared your own emotions by acknowledging and accepting them, new action would have been less likely. Change without awareness is like running blindfolded. When the blindfold of unaddressed emotion comes off and you know better the layout of your inner landscape, movement in new direction happens with confidence, not because you have to or should but because you can now see the way, and you innately want to go forward. So you do. You are driving.

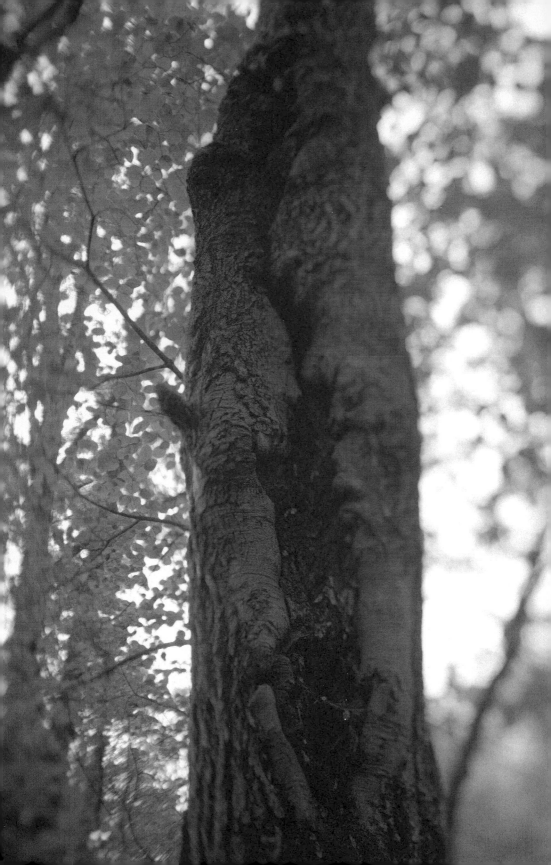

Chapter Seven

Flat Tires and Running Out of Gas: Treatment Alerts

*W*ell, you're making your way along the journey beyond diagnosis. You've started treatment or therapy. Or maybe you've had a tough but successful surgery. Congratulations. That shows courage. Entire books could be written documenting the remarkable effectiveness of our current medical practices. During your journey, like the path of so many, the process of treatment itself may have gone very well—uncomfortable at times, but that was expected.

And yet it is not uncommon during the treatment process to experience the unexpected. These surprises often let the air out of the tires of survivors, caregivers, and medical professionals. Many survivors have wished they had been informed of these possible flats. While perhaps uncomfortable to read, informing you is exactly what this chapter is designed to do.

This chapter first takes an honest look at some potential treatment surprises, describing those "flat tire" experiences in two categories: physical flat tires and emotional flat tires. We will end the chapter with a look at the issue of physical exhaustion—running out of gas. The intention in sharing the scenarios that follow is flat prevention; that is, to ready the reader for these possibilities and minimize negative psychological effects.

Physical Flat Tires

Consider an almost universal dread—needles. Many

treatments for illnesses involve the use of needles. Most people just don't like shots or needles, but it can come with the territory. Daily injections and even days of multiple sticks are not extraordinary. Those of us who have not had to go through daily "sticks" block out this part of the treatment process. Some survivors block the pain out too, especially when it's minor compared to other pains. But when you're in the midst of treatments by injection, the pain can be pretty hard to ignore—especially when complications set in. For instance, weakened veins that rupture can be messy and uncomfortable. This experience may flatten one of your tires. Some are surprised when their veins won't accept another needle; surprised when phlebotomists try lancing the top of the hand or foot.

But needles aren't the only source of physical flat tires on this journey. You might get a flat when a certain chemical or radiation treatment burns your skin or organs. Abdominal distress has flattened many tires. Appetites and taste buds can go flat with certain treatments. And what about drugs that treat your illness but also stimulate appetite? If you're having trouble eating, this is a wonderful thing. If eating isn't a problem, the weight gain may flatten a tire.

Others have treatment-related flats driving to the hospital. The familiar trip can set off anticipatory nausea. For some, this anticipatory discomfort happens when stepping into the hospital elevator or onto the treatment floor. Flat tires may result from impaired memory and concentration.

Steroids have ruined entire sets of tires. Many whose treatment regimens include steroids are completely unprepared for the mood swings often triggered, especially when the steroid dosage is cut back. Neuropathy—nerve damage that can result from certain chemical therapies—can bring loss of sensation and odd tingling in the hands or feet. More extensive cases are often painful and can make walking or use of the hands difficult. Usually, neuropathy subsides after treatment. Of course, this and any other physical flat tire may have *emotional* effects.

Emotional Flat Tires

Anyone who has been sick knows that emotions are often impacted by the illness. There is now clinical evidence that depression may be induced by some treatments for certain illnesses.[8] A psychiatrist from one of the country's leading hospitals supported this notion in sharing with me that some chemotherapies may exacerbate any anxiety and/or depression present in the survivor before treatment began.

Another emotional nail for flattening tires is that some survivors and caregivers are surprised when *they are asked to decide* which treatment option is best. There is justifiable litigation fear among many health care providers, making the journey beyond diagnosis sometimes more difficult for the survivors and the caregivers. And while treatment choices may help some consumers feel empowered, this same power is disconcerting for others who would prefer to have a physician express determined and overwhelming confidence in a treatment of choice.

Surgery patients have emotional flat tires when they see their bodies for the first time after the operation. Many say, "It's OK. I'm still alive," in the beginning.

Later, the sight of their scar(s) may make them feel sick, angry, or sad. Those in treatment soon after surgery may be surprised by how long it takes their incisions to heal. Another surprise can be the kind of pain felt, especially from certain shots that may produce deep muscle or bone discomfort.

Another emotional blowout for a lot of survivors is hair loss. There can be surprise when *all* body hair is lost. When this happens, it can feel like you lose something else: the one thing that kept you looking "normal." Now you are visibly "a patient" and, in some circles, everybody wants to talk with you about it. Sometimes that's great. Sometimes it's not. Either way, you lose some privacy. You lose the way people used to look at you. In different social or family settings, loss of hair can produce the opposite affect: People begin to avoid you—afraid of offending, not knowing what to say, afraid they might catch "it," or afraid of their own emotions.

A woman in a group once said, "I use to be Mary. Now I'm Cancer Mary." Illness seems to get between hugs and smiles and conversations. Consequently, there's what often feels like the steady erosion of a "normal" life. This can come with an emotional cost.

Running Out of Gas

As the treatments progress and these surprises take the air out of your tires, you may feel an energy loss, like you're running out of gas. Fatigue is believed by many to be the number one under-addressed treatment side effect for cancer. Of course, fatigue comes with many illnesses and treatments. In one study, 91 percent of the cancer survivors who experienced fatigue from chemo reported that the fatigue prevented a normal life. In that same study, of the patients who were employed before treatment, 75 percent changed their employment status because of fatigue. [9]

Treatment fatigue, for those of us who haven't felt it, cannot be comprehended. It's absolute exhaustion of all parts of the self: physical, emotional, mental, relational, and sometimes even spiritual. One may be too tired to read a paragraph or lift a glass of water, too tired to try to understand what is felt, too tired to pray or practice visualization, too tired to cry, too tired to know compassion for another, too tired to be anxious, too tired to move any part of the body.

What we have considered in this chapter is rough going. Perhaps you've recognized physical and emotional flat tires that you experienced during your treatment. Knowing that these same things have happened to others will hopefully ease your travels.

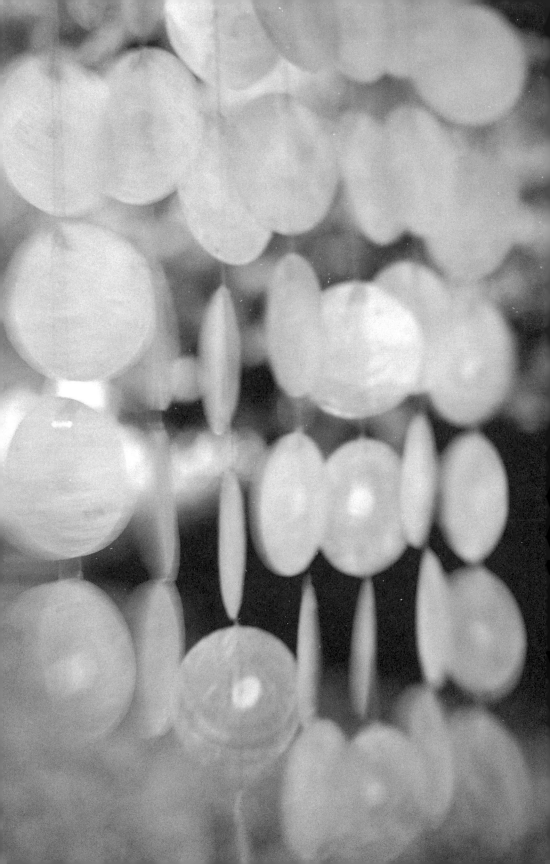

Chapter Eight

Rest Stop #2: One-Step Anxiety Management

At the last Rest Stop, ways to respond to emotions *in general* were discussed. This Rest Stop begins to address one specific emotion common on the journey beyond diagnosis: anxiety.

Speaking of the journey, have you had the pleasure of traveling with a four-legged friend? Did you bring your dog on this particular trip? Not a bad idea, given all we know about pet therapy. Ever notice what your dog does when it gets alarmed? Usually a dog will bark and then stand motionless without even breathing. We do the same thing. Watch. When something startles you, you freeze and stop breathing. At that moment, your whole system is receiving a message that says, "Warning! It's not safe. Don't relax. Don't trust. Be afraid. Be ready!" Oddly enough, it's a wonderful and primitive reaction that has preserved the species, because it initiates chemical changes in the body that make us more adept at managing physical threats.

When you hold your breath after being startled, the body floods your arms and legs with oxygen, producing a level of alertness, readiness, and tension throughout.

People sometimes get startled during the journey beyond diagnosis. However, there's evidence that *living* in this "alert" state can be costly, as the body holds the tension longer and longer. This prolonged startled experience becomes anxiety, and this state is especially troublesome for those who carried anxiety in their bodies even before the diagnosis.

An ongoing "it's not safe, don't relax, don't trust, be afraid, be ready" feeling can be truly exhausting. Fortunately, there is a way to interrupt this uncomfortable state. It's based on physiology. At a primitive level, the "alert" response *starts* when you hold your breath. For that reason, the breath becomes key to *interrupting* the building anxiety. Using this key, here's a **One-Step Anxiety Management** technique:

STEP 1: *Brrrrreeeeeaaaathe*

Actually, this one step has two parts: inhale and exhale. It's biology. When you stop breathing, you experience tension and "be afraid" feelings. When you breathe fully you invite relaxation and the "it's OK" feeling. Fear and trust are opposites, and the breath can be used to induce either. Short, rapid breaths or no breaths at all come with fear. Long, regular, full breaths come with trust. If you find yourself feeling anxious—experiencing those "don't relax, don't trust, be afraid, be ready" feelings—take fuller breaths. The body is hard wired to shift gears when you breathe fully. Deep breaths will help chase away the anxiety.

As we will explore in later chapters, it can be useful to notice fear and work with it rather than chase it away. But whenever you feel you need a quick fix, changing your breathing can provide that. (By the way, it would be good to begin the other exercises offered in this book with some of this conscious breathing.)

Now, if you're a two- or three-step kind of person, here's a second step to go along with the brrreeeaaathe step. Suggest the following thoughts to yourself as you breathe: "It's OK. In this moment, everything is all right."

And if you'd like a third step, here you go. Along with fuller breathing and "it's OK" thoughts, be aware of your legs and feet. Notice, for example, as you breathe deep, and think, "It's OK," how your feet feel against your socks or shoes. Through this practice you may start to sense more weight in your legs as your mind slows down and your anxiety eases. Combined, these tips might provide a quick way to feel a bit more comfortable on your journey, especially if you're anxious.

It should be noted that if you suffer from serious, persistent anxiety, professional help and/or medical intervention may be necessary.

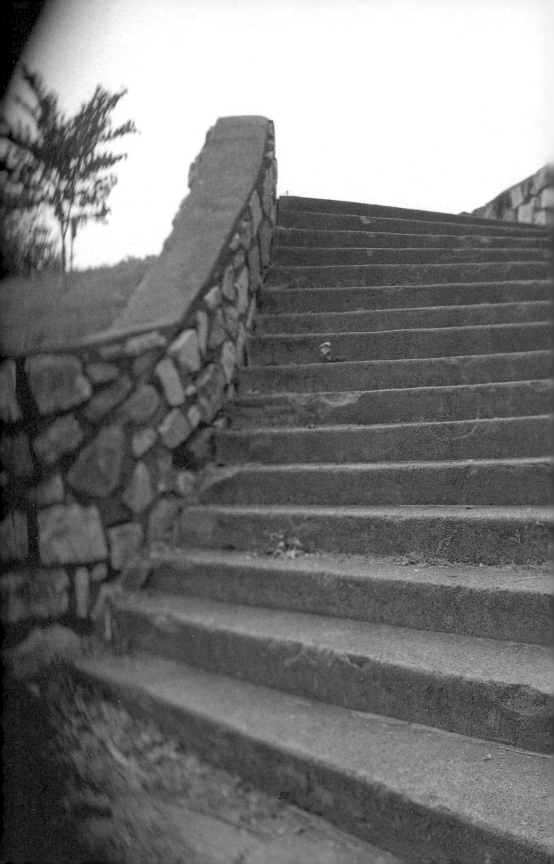

Chapter Nine

Detours: Matters that May Move You Off Your Recovery Road

So, you've been driving a while. And even though you may have had to change a flat tire or call Triple A for gas, you're following treatment protocols, dealing with side effects, responding to your emotions, and maybe even noticing moments that look, taste, and feel like some kind of normalcy. Yes. Experience these as fully as you like. Simply being aware of this goodness in your life does wonders. Take time to sample it often if that helps.

However, as with any long drive, sooner or later there may be detours. A detour is anything that takes you away from the direct path. The direct path for most survivors is recovery. Recovery may be physical, mental, emotional, relational, or even spiritual. Recovery could be all these. A detour is anything that commands your attention, time, or energy enough to impact the steadiness and strength of that recovery.

Detours of Family and Relationships

Detours on the journey beyond diagnosis come in many forms. Most common are family detours. If you are surviving an illness, having a spouse, partner, or primary support person become significantly ill can obviously be a detour. A troubled teenager is another possible detour. Repeated hospitalizations, extreme fatigue, or a scared child that constantly struggles with the survivor's appearance may all be detours.

Here are a few family detours of a different variety. A member of the family may decide to become the survivor's advocate, though one has not been requested. Consequently, the survivor may have to work hard, for example, at avoiding unwanted information about unsolicited reports of experimental treatments. In situations like this, the survivor or caregiver may need to draw a line, or focus more clearly on self care.

Bob was diagnosed with Parkinson's Disease and making his way as best he could, literally and emotionally. As his physical condition worsened, Bob's brother, Todd, began to call and e-mail several times a day. When Bob showed up for counseling, he spent as much time talking about his brother as he did himself.

"My brother's really angry," Bob reported. "I think he's having a harder time of this than me."

"What does that do to you, Bob?" I questioned.

"I need to keep my focus and keep my head on straight, but he's angry, and all his calls and questions are slowing me down," Bob answered.

As Bob got dialed into his own emotional experience, there was room for learning ways to stay separate from his brother's reactions. Unfortunately, Bob had to spend some of his resources on his brother's issues.

One detour that can be even more difficult is a family member deciding he or she knows what is best for the survivor. All of a sudden, the illness survivor is defending his or her actions to this person. This "I know best" detour can also impact the caregiver and the medical professional. Precious time and energy may be spent diverting this person's well-intentioned push. The expense is especially costly for the survivor.

Similarly, a spouse may decide that the doctor respected

by the survivor is not worth his or her weight in salt. Every doctor appointment becomes an inquisition. The survivor becomes more mediator than patient. If this kind of tension escalates, doctor appointments become trauma.

Oddly enough, another detour may be a spouse who feels jealous of the treatment process and all the attention the survivor is getting. Sounds strange, but it happens—and sometimes for perfectly understandable reasons. (Later, we will look closer at the journey beyond diagnosis from the caregiver's perspective.)

Finally, it often happens that survivors look fine but feel anything but. Consequently, others may expect the illness survivor to perform according to pre-disease standards. This may become a detour when someone important to the survivor believes the survivor is milking the situation and not pulling their weight.

Changes in the Medical Team as Detours

Changes in the makeup of the medical team can create detours. Survivors, caregivers, and medical professionals alike can struggle with the retirement, relocation, or death of key doctors, nurses, chaplains, social workers, or counselors. When everything else feels out of control, the constancy of the treatment team can hold many people together. I've heard survivors say that at times they feel more connected to their doctors and nurses than they do to their own families.

When, for whatever reason, a survivor has to separate from a trusted doctor or nurse, the loss can sting. This is a detour. Some survivors may choose to "fire" one doctor and "hire" another. While this is more choice, all the difficulty of moving medical records and establishing new relationships can be exhausting and a detour in its own right.

Other Detours

Did you notice? All the detours we've just discussed are *relationship detours.* But there are other kinds of detours. For example, severe and prolonged side effects may be an emotional detour. Having a job threatened in some way can be a detour. The matter of insurance is often a detour. Too many people stopping by for too many visits can be a detour. Folks telling you stories of all the people they know who died from your illness or the illness of your loved one may be a detour. Criticism for honest emotion or tears can be a detour. But all these pale in comparison to the most feared of all detours—recurrence. Recurrence of an illness is more than a detour for most survivors. It's a crash. For that reason, we will give it special attention in Chapter 19.

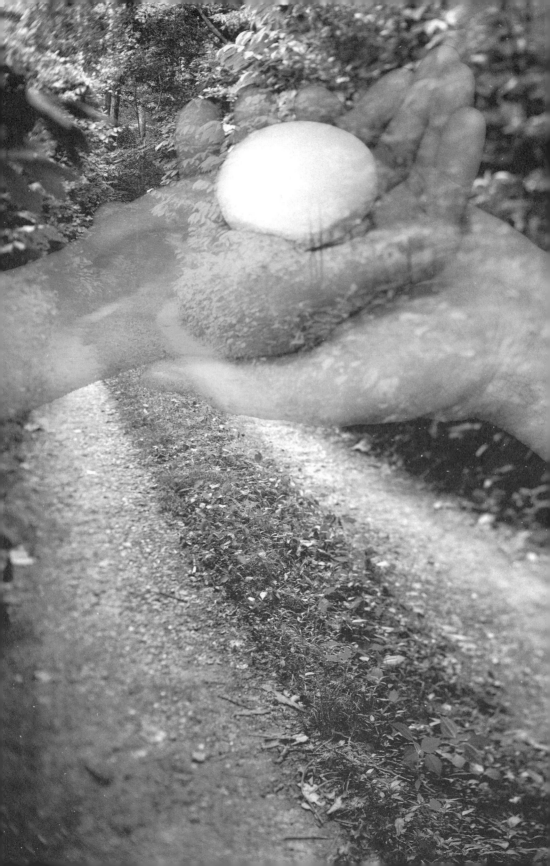

Chapter Ten

Travel Tips for Couples

*I*n the previous chapter, we talked about relationship changes, pressures, and detours. To circumvent as many of these detours as possible, when traveling *with someone* for a long time on the diagnosis journey, consider these tips.

For Caregivers

• As a survivor once said, *"If you don't got it, you don't get it."* In other words, if you haven't experienced a diagnosis, you really can't understand all that the survivor is going through. It usually doesn't help when you say you understand. Just be with the survivor when he or she needs you.

• Keep in mind that pain, fatigue, and treatments can affect everyone's moods. The survivor is not "herself/himself" mentally, physically, emotionally, relationally, or even spiritually. More often than not, it's best not to expect him or her to be. This expectation leads to frustration for everybody.

• Survivors in treatment can experience kindness like medicine, and unkindness like salt in wounds.

• **D.A.A.A. = Don't assume anything—ask.** Don't assume that the survivor needs to be cheered on. Don't assume that he or she doesn't. Don't assume that the survivor needs to feel hopeful today. Don't assume that he or she doesn't. Don't assume that the survivor needs to eat more, exercise more, sleep more, or have more sex. Don't assume that he or she doesn't. Don't assume that the survivor needs your company or conversation. Don't assume that he or she doesn't. Instead of assuming, ask the simple question, "What can I do for you right now that would be most helpful?" And remember, what is needed right now could change in less than an hour.

• Did you know that when you tell everyone you see that the survivor (your spouse, friend, lover, or patient) "handles this so well," or "always has a great sense of humor, even with the pain," or "never complains," you may be sending the message to that survivor, "I need you to be strong?" So who then is going to be strong for the survivor? Where is the survivor supposed to go with the tough feelings that naturally occur?

• Did you know that by repeatedly telling someone who is physically hurting, "You look great," you may be discounting that person's pain? On the other hand, when people in pain (physical or emotional) are simply listened to, their pain often decreases, and tough emotions dissipate more quickly.

• Caregivers, you may not have a diagnosed illness, but you do have the same rights as the survivor. Yes, you're going to give the survivor more leeway, but don't give yourself away in the process. Don't let yourself be taken advantage of. That's not good for anybody. In taking care of yourself, it's OK to say things like, "Look, I know you're exhausted and frustrated, but when I do something by myself you seem to get upset."

• A time may come (often after treatment ends) when you want to act like nothing ever happened. For the short run, that attitude may get you through. And such an approach does seem to work for some through the long haul. But something did happen. The mental, emotional, physical, relational, and spiritual ramifications of that "something" can be significant. *Never* allowing yourself to visit *any* of those affected parts may take a toll.

• The person diagnosed is busy taking care of himself/herself. You're responsible for you. It's very important that you maintain your own health and well-being. A 2002 study in *Health Psychology* reported that chronic illness in a partner may negatively affect the caregiver's physical and mental health.[10]

For Survivors

• The person supporting you probably loves you. He or she wants so much to take your pain away—wants so much to help. Your caregiver really doesn't know what you're going through. Don't expect that. Your caregiver is not a mind reader. Don't expect that either. When you tell your caregiver what you need, you help that person avoid making assumptions, and you're more likely to get what's important to you.

• Your caregiver may find it difficult to leave you or do things that are good for him or her. However, if your caregiver doesn't respect his or her own needs, you will both live in the resentment that builds. If you're currently homebound, earnestly encourage your caregiver to take time for himself or herself. Invite someone else in to stay with you if you need that. You have to be loving but firm about this if you really want your caregiver to stay well. You'll both benefit from it.

• As the survivor, it's possible that you feel powerless. You may feel as if you have very little control of your emotions or the illness. Consequently, you may be looking for something or someone to control as a way to make yourself feel better—as a way to feel some sense of mastery in this difficult situation. Many times the person you try to control is the person closest to you. This can look like nitpicking, like nothing that person does is right. **Remember, you are not the only one with needs.**

• A time may come (often after treatment ends) when you want to act like nothing ever happened. For the short run, that attitude may get you through. And such an approach does seem to work for some through the long haul. But something did happen. The mental, emotional, physical, relational, and spiritual ramifications of that "something" can be significant. *Never* allowing yourself to visit *any* of those affected parts may take a toll.

• Finally, your courage and heroism may uplift many people. That can be wonderful. But if you never say *no* as the survivor, take a break, or let others know what you need in a direct way, resentment can build in you. Your caregiver will likely become the target of that anger. Always saying yes and rarely saying no may be a way of life that is difficult to undo. Chapter 21 offers special sections on this subject, along with suggestions on learning to say no.

For Survivors and Caregivers

Accept one another where you are, not where you think the other should be. Out of your own need, you may give love only when the person you're on the journey with hits the mark you have deemed the gold standard: "There's that great smile." Obviously, this statement could be sending the message, "If you, my love, are not happy on the outside all the time, you're letting me down." This can burden the heart.

Next, be mindful of who and how many you tell

about the illness. If one of you doesn't want the whole world to know, the other would be wise to support that. Yes, a community of caring people that knows about the illness can and often does make the journey easier for both the survivor and the caregiver. However, folks can do funny things with the news of your situation. They can one-up you—tell stories of someone with the same kind of illness who had the same treatments but more difficult side effects. Their emotion can drain your emotion.

Not only that, when it comes to numbers of people who "know," there may be a point of diminishing return. If everywhere you go, people ask about the illness, you might feel trapped—no place to be free from all that the illness experience carries. Many survivors have told me that they just want to be treated normally. This isn't denial. There are just times they don't want to go there. It is nice to have some surroundings that are "illness free" or people who don't know. When you're there or with them for just a little bit, the illness isn't — like maybe at a book club or exercise class. That can be a relief.

Sex and Cancer

This is a couple's topic, and one I would be remiss not to address. What I'm about to share was learned from survivors and their loved ones. It's second hand, but I think it deserves to be said. Keep in mind, I am not a sex therapist. If you have serious medical questions about this subject, talk with your doctor or nurse. Social workers are also helpful with these matters.

For some men and women in treatment, the sex life

barely skips a beat. These people can both satisfy and be satisfied by their mates. For a lot of others, things aren't that simple.

In the beginning, having sex doesn't even make it on the top-ten list for many. In time, however, the physically intimate part of relationship gains strength as a need. Often the need of one partner is not matched by the need of the other. Strong couples manage this well. And yet a diagnosis can wreak havoc on even the surest marriages and relationships. Someone has to take the initiative and bring to light whatever is not getting talked about.

It's not uncommon for women in treatment to experience vaginal dryness, making sexual intercourse extremely uncomfortable. Estrogen-based creams compound the problem for women in treatment for certain cancers. Talk to your doctor about other lubricant options. Radiation to any part of the body, if the skin has been burned, can make sexual contact difficult. It's like trying to make love when you have a sunburn.

Obviously, surgery to any part of the body requires healing time. When the body is tender in any place, pain becomes a distraction to sexual satisfaction. This is especially true when areas near the breasts or genitals are affected.

It's not uncommon for men in certain treatments to have erectile dysfunction. And while some men are OK for a while sharing physical intimacy with their mates in non-intercourse ways, that may lose its charm. Men often feel "less-than" if they aren't able to satisfy or be satisfied by their mates through intercourse, even if the mate reports that it isn't important. Moreover, not being able to have an orgasm frustrates many men. Women feel that same frustration. Both partners can feel diminished when too tired or unable to either satisfy or be satisfied. This can feed any depression that may be present, which itself can weaken libido.

All this can put a dent in self-esteem. When you factor in the potential loss of self-worth that often accompanies loss of professional performance, or the perceived loss of effectiveness as a parent or spouse, the self could take a serious hit. This lowered esteem may circle back to limit sexual drive, "performance," and/or satisfaction.

Women and men left with scars may be especially sensitive to being seen unclothed. This can be disarming to their mates. You usually can't go wrong by gently and lovingly opening this issue for pillow talk, wrapped in lots of acceptance.

Lovers also get confused by when, what, and how to touch. There is uncertainty about what feels good and what may actually hurt. There is uncertainty about whether the lack of interest in sex is a product of physical discomfort or a reflection of the relationship. When one partner initiates, the other may be confused by recent history. Is this a sign that my lover wants to get closer, or is it going to pass? Does my mate want more contact or more time? Is this a hug thing, or something more?

And don't expect all this to change when treatment is successfully completed. First of all, if treatment has impacted sexual function, it may not return as soon as treatment stops. Patience with each other at times like these will help a lot. All these questions are great topics of discussion. Don't wait until you find yourself in a situation of sexual uncertainty. Talk about it over dinner or sometime before you lie down. Remember not to assume anything. It's a good way to prevent hurt feelings.

Finally, intimacy is more than intercourse, and intimacy is not just physical. Whether you and your mate are discussing intimacy or IV therapy, *respect* may be the most helpful element of all. And respect may be best demonstrated by just listening. Silence is golden. It's also an art, and perhaps the most important of travel tips. How many of you, when telling someone close to you about the diagnosis, were offered pure silence? Silence, artfully presented, communicates the deepest respect for what the speaker may be thinking and feeling. People often don't hear until they've been heard.

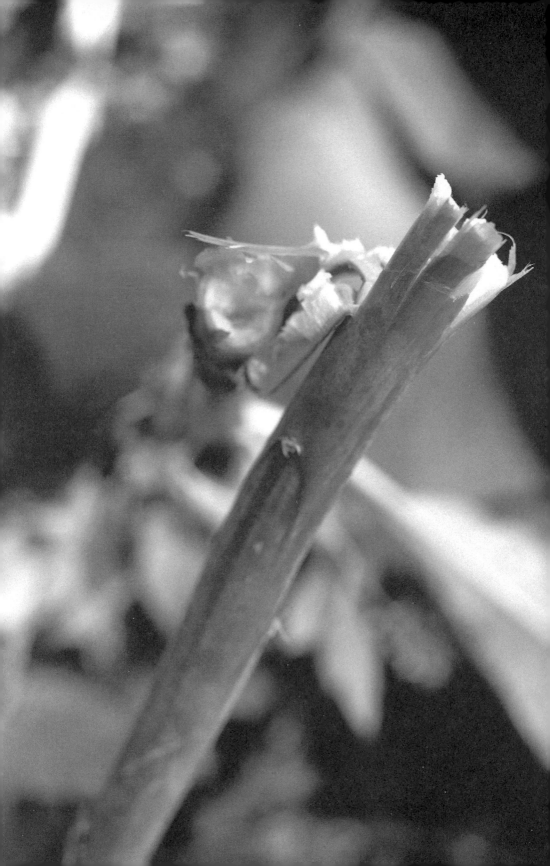

Chapter Eleven

Rest Stop #3:
Stress Bustin'

ost trips have their stressful moments. Many would say this is especially true with the journey beyond diagnosis. Some basic stress management information could be useful for this sojourn.

So far, we have talked off and on about both anxiety and stress. We've defined anxiety—but what exactly is stress? Well, if you think of the stress you have had during your own illness, you will likely discover there was something you wanted at that stressful time that you weren't getting. You wanted peace, you wanted health, you wanted to see your child graduate, but you felt your illness would interfere with getting one or all of those. This begins to define stress. Stress equals experiencing a block in front of something you want: **S**tress = **B**lock x **W**ant, or **S** = **B x W**. The multiplication sign suggests that the more blocks you feel, the more stress.

Stress **B**ustin' is really about **Ch**oice: **SB = Ch**. And it's not so much about what you choose but *that* you choose. This is all about finding and living with your power. Are you aware of how many choices you've made in the last twelve hours? You decided what time to get up. Most likely, you decided to get up with someone next to you or to sleep alone. You did. Nobody put a gun to your head and said, "Get up." Nobody forced you to marry your spouse or is forcing you to live alone. "Well," you may say, "nobody put a gun to my head to make me get up, but if I didn't get up, I would be late for work." OK, so you chose to get up to be on time. "Well," you might say, "I have to be on time, or I'll lose my job." OK, so you have chosen to keep your job.

The idea is, when we live fully in the awareness of our choices, our life comes alive. We start to see it as self-created rather than imposed. Yow. When you press this issue, you realize that everything you have is exactly what you want. Wait, before you slam the book shut hear me out. Think about it. If what you have isn't what you want, why don't you have something else? This isn't about blame. I'm not trying to make you feel bad. The intention is liberation.

Not only that. If you find yourself feeling uncomfortable as you read this, in a way you are fortunate. The discomfort is trying to tell you something. Not everyone is willing to hear that discomfort. Consequently, for those that don't hear, things don't change.

I shared this "We have what we want or we'd have something else" concept with a group of teachers. A woman in the crowd who had been restless in her chair for a while finally stood up and proclaimed, "My husband left me with three kids. The youngest is this big. Do you think this is what I want?"

I said, "You know, I read last winter about a woman who left a baby in a gym bag in the dead of winter in a city park. You could do that."

She snapped, "I've been sitting here thinking you were crazy. Now I know you are. I would never do that!"

"Exactly," I said. "You would never do that because what you want is to love and value your children so they will feel loved and valued in life. You are choosing to stay for that reason, as hard as it may be." Nobody was making her raise those kids. As long as she was willing to deal with the consequences, she too could walk.

She really could. What she had was a choice, and through the discussion she began to see what she was choosing. When she really understood this notion, she changed. Her body language totally shifted. She tasted a tinge of freedom then.

A final story about choice: A guy came up to me after a presentation for store managers from around the country. Briefcase in hand he said, "Greg, that stuff about stress bustin' is all fine and good, but you know what would really take care of my stress: a johnboat, a six-pack, and the Florida Keys. I live in a stinkin' town, with a mortgage as big as my neighborhood and a truckload a' kids. The only thing that's gonna touch my stress is The Keys."

"So why don't you go upstairs, make a few calls, and go?" I asked. He looked at me like I was nuts. "Yeah," I said, "Call your family, pack up the works, and go. Who's stoppin' you? Now, you may be out there fishing one day, and some guys paddle up in suits saying, 'Hi, we're from Visa,' but if you're willing to deal with that, go!"

He looked at me for a second, then cocked his head like a pup. He got it. Nobody was making him live in a stinking town. Nobody was making him stay in his job or his house, or his marriage for that matter. When he got the power of his past, present, and future choices, something lifted from him. He understood that what he had was what he must want, or he'd have something else. The same is true for each of us.

"What about my house being struck by lightning?" "What about my child getting MD?" These are, of course, external circumstances over which we have no control. This is not about hurting anyone or making anyone feel responsible for these terribly painful situations. In the human mind, we would never choose to have a house get struck by lightning or ourselves or anyone we love be afflicted with a difficult circumstance or illness.

And yet, even within these, there are choices. I kept a little sign on my bulletin board for years that read: "Sometimes all we may have control of is where we place our attention."

The simple act of recognizing choice eases most situations. The freedom is not so much in making different choices, but in knowing you have, do, and will choose. Your life is not imposed. Situations or events may feel imposed. How you respond is never imposed.

The Three-Step Stress Bustin' Process

Step 1. Identify what you want
Step 2. Ask yourself, "Is this worth having?"
Step 3. Choose

Step 1. Identify What You Want

Say you feel stressed during the holidays because thoughts pop into your mind that this holiday may be your last. If you are very, very sick, these can be very real thoughts, and so are the feelings that come along. You might find the last four chapters of this book useful now. But let's assume that you have a very positive prognosis and check-ups over the last three years have been good. And what you would like is to feel something other than stress at the next holiday.

So, if we break this down using the stress equation described earlier, the stress (S) is anxiety during the holidays. What you want (W) might be peace of mind or more relaxation. The block (B) is a nagging thought that you may not have another holiday with the people you love.

Step 2. Ask Yourself, "Is This Worth Having?"

So, Step 1 is about recognizing what it is that you want. Step 2 is about evaluating whether or not what you want is really worth having.

Go back to wanting more peace of mind. It seems pretty obvious. In answer to the Step 2 question, "Is this worth having?" how could peace of mind ever not be worth having? Well, here's one way. What if your spouse had a persistent pain in the lower abdomen? And what if that spouse decided on peace of mind, in spite of the pain? That's great, and it is possible. Some people are able to achieve great peace in the face of pain through mental exercise.

But what if the lack of peace was a message from your spouse's body to take action and look into the pain? Peace of mind in this case may not be "worth it" since ignoring the pain could prove harmful.

Try a different example to get us through Step 2. What if you're stressed because your teenage daughter refuses to tell you how she feels about your diagnosis? The stress (S) is your ongoing concern that she is holding everything in. What you want (W) is for her to express herself to you. What's the block (B) here? Could it be your relationship with her? Could it be your belief that she needs to talk about your diagnosis with you? She could be talking with her friends as a way of protecting you from her feelings. Is her expressing herself to you worth having? Maybe it is. Maybe it isn't.

Step 3. Choose

Once you've gotten clear about what you want and decided it really is worth having, Step 3 suggests you make choices to get it. Back to the example of wanting to feel more relaxed during the holidays: Say you think it is worthwhile to feel more relaxed, and a holiday is upon you. Having made that choice, what will you do to bring more relaxation about? Will you learn some anxiety management techniques? Good. What if you decide that trying to address the holiday anxiety right now is going to eat up the precious energy you believe you need just to get through the holiday? So be it. Maybe you'll choose to put fear out of mind at this time, not because you just want to ignore it, but because you've decided leaving it alone right now is best. All right. You get to choose.

And that's the power of Stress Bustin'—living fully conscious of the power you have to choose, every minute, every day. That awareness about choice is life-giving. While the actions you choose are important, the awareness that you *can* choose is more important. You are not powerless about the stress.

A quick look back at the example of the teenager who won't talk: Say you decide that it is important for you and your daughter to talk. You have been watching her, and she seems depressed: grades are slipping, she spends a lot of time alone, she looks ill. OK, so what will you choose to do about that? Maybe you'll start with a phone call to the school counselor, or speak at length about it with your spouse to figure out how to respond as parents. Good. Or maybe you'll decide that you can't spend a lot of effort on this circumstance right now. In a few weeks, maybe, when your strength is back. Good. So when your daughter continues to hide her feelings, you see it, but instead of getting stressed, you recognize the choice you have made to let it go for now. While acting so cleanly on these kinds of decisions isn't as simple as one, two, three, the more you practice the power of choice, the more fluid it all becomes.

It's not about right or wrong. It's about choice. It's about living fully aware that so much of your life (even if it's only your inner life) is a product of your choices. Such a life is much different from the emotional, mental, or even spiritual life that feels imposed by someone or something else. Living in awareness of choice lowers stress. Life gets better.

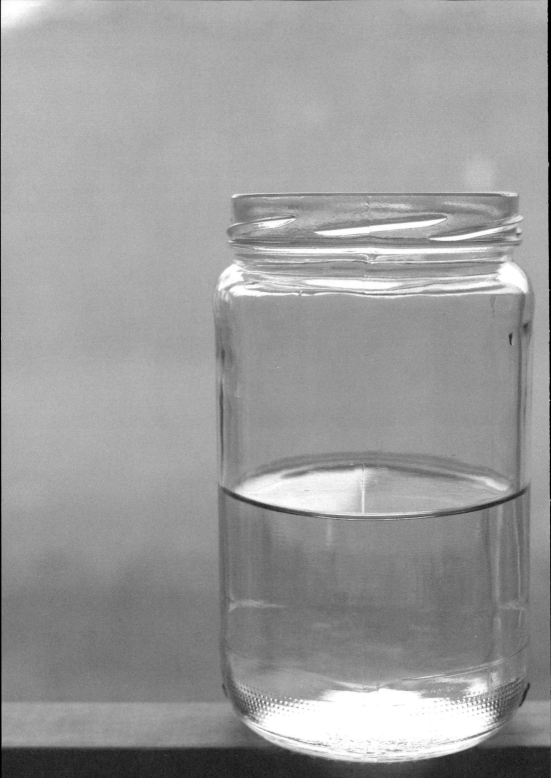

Chapter Twelve

Mountaintops: Seeing Life from a New Perspective

D o you know what it's like to drive through a beautiful landscape, climb to elevated terrain, and look back? The view from these higher heights can make things look different and even better. Illness can do the same to your perceptions of life.

Hundreds of survivors, caregivers, and medical professionals alike report that life is not the same once you've journeyed beyond diagnosis. Life has more meaning. Simple things matter more. Some say they take better care of themselves. They've learned to say no. Some feel little concerns bother them less. Some say they found their voice and speak up now. Many find peace and improved marriages.

Many explain how their values have shifted since being diagnosed. "There's more to life than work," many report. Consequently, they spend less time in the office. Some find their hearts and cry. Others are visited by compassion for all who suffer. In still others, something within pops open and joy comes out.

Some discover for the first time who they really are. Trauma has a way of sculpting off all that is not real so only the truth survives. Some let another's love in for the first time. From that moment on, such people allow a deep and powerful love to spring up inside.

Sometimes, one traveler changes in ways their mate can't or won't. In other travelers, great pools of hurt, sadness, or anger are uncovered. But fortified by the strength required to best the disease, sojourners on the illness journey dive into these turbulent waters, swimming for the solid shore of greater wholeness. And from these waters a new person is born. Like natural birth: first there's discomfort, then pain, then great pain, then birth, new life and real joy.

And from the high ground of an illness diagnosis, things may look very different. It's funny that when the self changes, even one's god can seem different. I am convinced that going through serious illness is some of the deepest work for a soul. Later chapters will explore this more closely. Suffice it to say that serious illness appears to open a window somewhere in the spirit of a person. Some climb through to a new land. Others don't. So be it. There is meaning in each way.

And then there's a second aspect of mountain climbing, and this, for me, is a delicate subject. Without care, anyone can fall from high places. There can be an emotional high from surviving any trauma. The line between a richly improved life and an unhealthy emotional high is thin.

"Loose Gravel!": If you've driven or hiked mountain passes, you've seen this sign. It's posted to protect travelers, which is exactly why these thoughts are offered in this chapter.

Surely you've met those who seem hollow with survivor high. Their joy is fragile. Their focus is narrow, so they might not see the loose rocks. The "drug" of the newfound self might only be another anesthesia against the old pain still unplowed deep in the belly of these dear people. In this fervor, they may find it difficult to tolerate any experience or worldview different from the one they now clutch. Consequently, distance can be created between them and those who really love them—those who can help them climb down safely.

Here's an example of how this dangerous climbing may appear. When I walked into the support group room, I saw Bonnie for the first time. She had an unsteady smile. Most new group members do. But hers was different. It held more than the usual discomfort that comes with meeting a new group of people under the circumstances of illness. I was immediately aware that her voice was carrying over most of the other group members as they chatted before we got started. It was hard not to notice the forceful quality of speech behind Bonnie's words. Entering the group room, I caught pieces of what she was saying, "And if you don't completely believe you're going to get better, you won't."

Our custom with new members to the weekly groups was to let them introduce themselves last. This helped take the pressure off new members, as they witnessed others introduce themselves. We also made sure that, as the last one to introduce him or herself, the new member could then take as much time as needed on this first day.

Bonnie seemed uneasy as she listened to others "tell their story." Seasoned group members, along with their introductions, often updated the group on their weeks. This included comments like, "I also found out I have to get additional testing done, and I'm pretty scared. I'd like to talk about this more after introductions."

The closer it got to Bonnie's turn for an introduction, the more uncomfortable she seemed, twisting on the edge of her seat and looking at her watch, purse still in hand. "This just doesn't have a good feeling to me. . . . Oh, my name is Bonnie," was her introduction. "I *had* breast cancer. I was diagnosed three weeks ago," she blurted. "I don't have it anymore. Surgery got rid of it, and I am doing all I can to stay well," beginning to shake as the words fell out.

"I'm afraid you are all very negative," Bonnie shuttered. "I heard people talking about being sad. And someone said they were afraid. I'm not. I am going to beat this. . . . I mean I have beaten this," she restated. She wrestled with the tears coming to her eyes but couldn't allow them as she said, "We can all beat this, but you have to be more hopeful. I'll stay and see how I feel, but this group may not be for me."

Group members were reacting to Bonnie. Some of the new people were picking up her angst and beginning to twist, too. The more mature group members simply sat with openness to Bonnie, and openness to their own feelings and reactions. Those somewhere between looked to me. Seasoned members knew it was tough starting in the group, so an experienced member spoke up: "Bonnie, being new to a group like this can be pretty uncomfortable. What would be most helpful to you right now?"

"I don't know. Can somebody say something good?" she responded.

"I remember my first day with the group," offered another group member. "I was the only one with kidney cancer and wondered if I would be able to connect to anyone else."

A male group member spoke up: "Yeah, I had a hard time with all this emotional stuff, but now I wouldn't miss the group for anything."

At that, Bonnie jumped up and shot to the door saying, "I can't do this. God bless you all. I love you. Please be happy." That was the last time we saw Bonnie. She did exactly what she needed to do. On the one hand, I accepted her reaction, but on the other, I felt sure that the powerful pain just below the surface for Bonnie would soon break through, and the group wouldn't be there to support her when it did.

Many people climb high into the mountains of survivorship, whether diagnosed or caregiver. Many make there way down, safe and sound. For those still climbing, please pay attention to the signs.

Mountaintops and scenic overviews are a precious part of the journey beyond diagnosis for all who travel. Enjoy the beauty along the high roads. Be careful to come down. The groundedness you'll find in the foothills—in the honesty of *all* that you feel—will make for a real and "whole-ly" way of life.

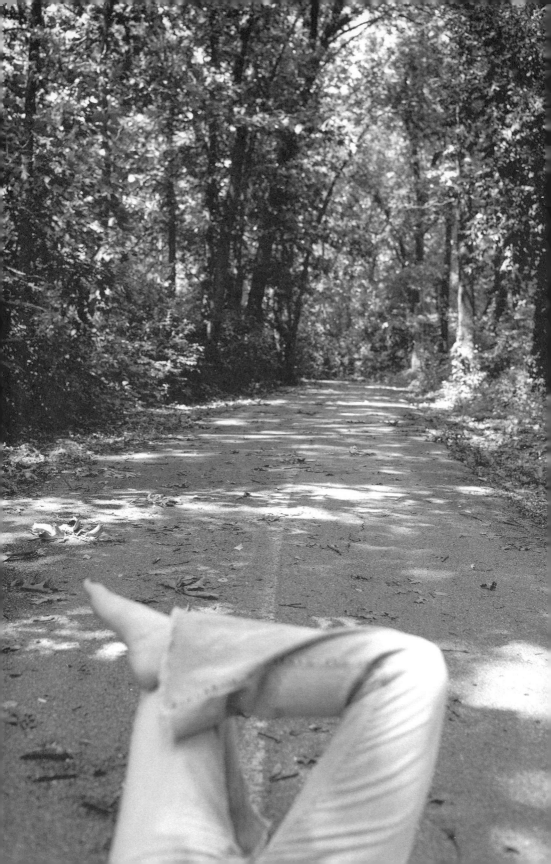

Chapter Thirteen

Rest Stop #4: Values and Voting with Your Feet

ave you ever pulled off at a rest stop just to think? That's what this rest stop is all about: considering your values. The expression, "You vote with your feet" certainly paints an interesting picture. It's also true. The idea is that your values are better represented by your *actions* than by your *words*.

The exercise in this chapter helps you gain awareness of your vote. Let the exercise inform you. It's for your eyes only. Be genuine with your responses and you'll get more out of it. If you find that what you say about your values matches your actions, great. That is very good for you. You probably have, more or less, what you want in your life.

If you find that what you say about your values does not match your actions, great. That is very good for you. You will then perhaps know which actions to take to make your life feel better. Taking these actions, freely and by choice, will make you feel more like you have what you want in your life. And that may improve your life's quality, and that is enough. But if your quality of life gets better, so may your health.

There's no right or wrong about your responses to this exercise. It's just information. Let the information speak to you in its own way. There is no score comparing here, just a chance to increase your awareness.

Step 1.   Take Some Time.   Make a List of the Ten Things You Value Most

Give this a minute. Try to zero in on the top ten most important features, actions, people, practices, beliefs, etc., in your life today. This can be anything: your family, your faith, your exercise plan, your financial plan, your time, your breakfast, your doctor, your dog, your job, your diary, beauty, serenity, anything.

Step 2. Prioritize Your List

When you're ready, list the ten items you came up with in rank order down the left side of a sheet of paper with the most important item from your list at the top of the sheet and the least important item at the bottom of the sheet. Feel free to use the form at the end of this chapter.

Step 3. Make Five Columns with the Following Headings:
> *How Often*
> *How Long*
> *How Much*
> *Feeling*
> *Give Up*

To create the columns, draw five lines about an inch apart down your sheet to the right of the prioritized list of your ten most important items. Write the five headings shown above across your sheet, one on the top of each column.

Step 4. Rate Your Original Top Ten List Under Each Heading

Here are the meanings of each heading:

How Often: How regularly do you engage in this feature? Put the number 10 in this column beside the feature from your original top-ten list that you do the most often. Put the number 1 in this column beside the feature from your list that you do the least often. If you listed beauty, for example, on your original list, how often do you find it, or how often do you create experiences that expose you to beauty? If, in this way, you experience beauty more often than you do any other thing from your list, then put the number 10 beside "Beauty" under the column, "How Often." If you put tennis on your list, and you play a lot, but not as often as you experience beauty, then you would put the number 9 beside tennis.

How Long: When you do engage in this feature, how much time do you spend? Put the number 10 in this column beside the feature from your list of ten that you spend the most time with. Put the number 1 in this column beside the feature from your list that you spend the least time with.

How Much: When you do engage in this feature, how much does it cost? Prioritize your list in the same way you did under the first two headings, i.e., 10 beside the item that costs the most, etc.

Feeling: When you do engage in this feature, how good does it make you feel? Put the number 10 in this column beside the feature from your list of ten that makes you feel the best, etc.

Give Up: Which of the ten features from your list would you most willingly give up? Put the number 10 in this column beside the feature from your list that you would be *least* willing to give up completely. Put the number 1 in this column beside the feature from your list that you would be *most* willing to give up completely.

Finally, total all the numbers to the right of each of your original ten important items. So, do you vote with your feet? If this column of totals is highest at the top, decreases as it goes down the page, and is lowest at the bottom, then you do vote with your feet. If it doesn't, then your actions suggest those things that are most important to you have the higher totals to the right, and those things that are least important to you have the lower totals to the right.

What's most important about this exercise is that it offers you a chance to discover more of what you really value. The purpose is simply to invite you to pay more attention to the people, places, experiences, and beliefs that bring you life. Refresh yourself.

Vote with Your Feet

YOUR TOP TEN ITEMS BELOW	How Often?	How Long?	How Much?	Feeling?	Give Up?	Total Points
1						
2						
3						
4						
5						
6						
7						
8						
9						
10						

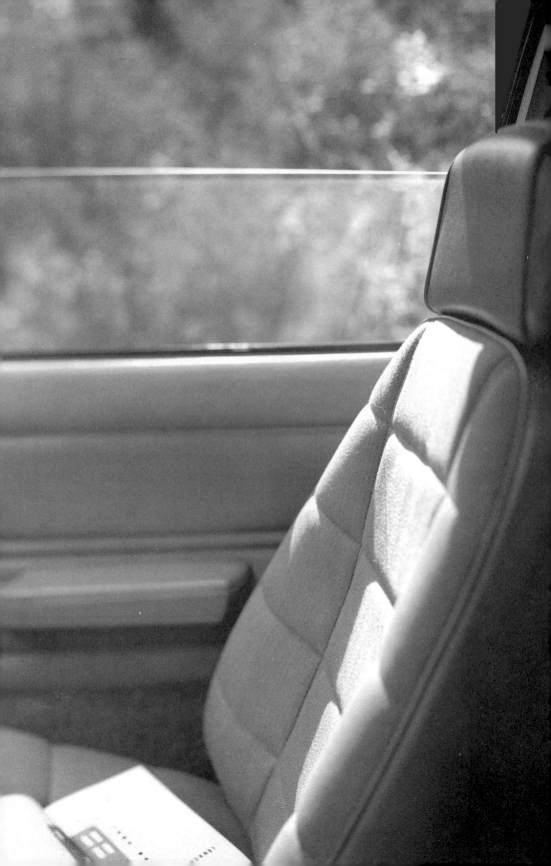

Chapter Fourteen

Who's Really Driving: View from the Caregiver's Window

*E*verybody on the journey beyond diagnosis needs refreshments, regardless of who's driving, since anyone closely involved with an illness survivor can be deeply affected by the travel. This chapter speaks to those taking the journey *with* the illness survivor, especially as primary caregivers.

Susan's best buddy, her father, was told he had a rare form of salivary gland cancer. Because she had decided to leave town to be with her dad, Susan came to group for the last time.

"My dad's fighting this illness with all his might," she spoke through her tears. "He's throwing punches, and taking punches, bleeding, and down on one knee. And all I can do is stand in the corner and hold the towel." This, probably better than any explanation, describes what it's like to be a primary caregiver for someone on the journey beyond diagnosis. It aptly represents the sense of utter helplessness shared by so many caregivers. And yet, given the gravity of the survivor's circumstance, this weight carried by the caregiver often goes unnoticed.

For caregivers, this poignancy is felt day to day, if not moment to moment. And with the added responsibilities that often accompany the caregiver role, caregivers may find themselves asking the question, "Who is really driving? Now I'm not only responsible for groceries, laundry, kids, and the lawn, but finances, doctor appointments, and the extended family. Now I'm counselor, newly defined lover, nurse, and provider, just to name a few."

Behind the scenes, the caregiver may be running interference with family members and coworkers of the survivor. Caregivers may also have discreet discussions with the medical community. And it's this fine line between these facets of caregiving and the survivor's need for self-governance where things can get a little dicey.

For example, maybe the survivor has sent the message early and clearly that he or she wants to do all the driving. He or she wants to be the point person for all treatments, and schedules, and communications with doctors and nurses. And while survivors do the very best they can, since their concentration, strength, and memory may be affected by the illness or the treatments, they sometimes miss things. On days like this, caregivers feel a bit handcuffed. They don't want to undermine the control the survivor may be clutching too, but they also don't want unnecessary harm or pain to visit the survivor. So, while it may be unclear who's really driving, the caregiver gently takes hold of the wheel.

Here's what it looks like from the caregiver's window. Caregivers get tired, but they are less likely to acknowledge it. There are certain feelings caregivers reveal only to other caregivers. For example, caregivers often feel devalued. How many times has a couple dealing with illness gone out only to have everyone ask the survivor, "How are you?" without any recognition of the caregiver's pain.

Caregivers think ESP is critical for effectively doing the job, but they don't have it. They can't read the survivor's mind. Caregivers believe they have just found the right thing to say, the right food to prepare, or the right way to hold the survivor, and boom, just like that, it changes. All this supports the caregiver's nagging sense of helplessness.

Caregivers may doubt the strength of the survivor's love for them and their love for the survivor. Most work this out, but we all know couples that haven't. A diagnosis, for many, is the most forceful pressure endured in a relationship. And yes, many caregivers wish *they* had been diagnosed with the illness. On the other hand, caregivers sometimes wish it was over. That is, in especially painful and prolonged treatment protocols, caregivers can catch themselves wishing the survivor would die and end the physical, emotional, mental, and spiritual pain. But if one half of a couple is thinking these thoughts, the other probably is, too. In a strong relationship, even such tough thoughts are brought to light, and the darkness felt by caregiver and survivor lifts a bit.

❖ ❖ ❖

Caregivers don't know how much to push and how much to be patient. I've heard many survivors tell that if it wasn't for their mates giving them a solid nudge once in a while, they wouldn't have made it. On the other hand, many survivors wish people would just back away. Trying to find this balance takes its toll on caregivers. Caregivers fight with God. Unfortunately, God doesn't fight back, and they end up feeling profoundly alone.

While it's essential for caregivers to take care of themselves, they often feel lost in the treatments, moods, and twenty-four-hour-a-day care provision. Caregivers forget who they really are. They have morphed so many times to the situation at hand that they feel unanchored in a personality. What often comes before this loss of self is the use of historically effective responses to a crisis. But now, nothing seems to be working. This can be followed by a surrender in the caregiver. Such letting go can be power-fully good. It can be a window for growth. However, it is usually also powerfully painful and confusing.

Caregivers forget to send the bill, turn off the stove, take the kids, or fix the door. But remembering is on their "to do" list. Caregivers expect themselves to be strong, to hold the survivor up. It's not always this way, but usually. It is part of our culture to focus away from ourselves when someone we love is in real need. Thank goodness for this "instinct." It works wonderfully, to a point.

Caregivers and survivors both know this "point," when selflessness stops working. This breaking point usu-ally comes when a treatment rhythm is established, long after preliminary tests, procedures, and surgeries are done. This point—when caregiver selflessness wears thin—may arrive when treatments go on and on. It may show up when the survivor (in the caregiver's opinion) is having a hard time moving on with his or her life. We are talking about the point when everybody's nerves are cooked. The caregiver can't hold back his or her feelings another min-ute, and can't wait on the survivor one more time. You get the picture. However, this point is often not reckoned with.

One way to avoid reaching this breaking point is for the caregiver to begin to acknowledge, accept, and act on his or her own needs, not just the needs of the survivor. Actually, the sooner the caregiver is able to do this respect-fully, the better.

I was discussing this point on a TV show when the interviewer said, "But Greg, don't you think the survivor is saying, 'Look, I'm the one with the illness. I'm the one going through treatments. I have a right to be taken care of, no matter what. For better or for worse, in sickness and in health.'" I said, "Yep, and the caregiver has a right to have boundaries."

It's not an "either/or." It's one of those "boths." If the caregiver doesn't take care of him or herself, tremendous resentment will build. If you, as a caregiver, feel resentment, take a good look at how well a job you're doing of taking care of yourself. First of all, there's a good chance your resentment will lessen when you mobilize your own needs. Do something about them.

Secondly, if you really want to do the best for the one you're caring for, take care of yourself, too. Don't think for a second that your resentment is not experienced in every tone, touch, word, and gesture you offer. And what's also important is the fact that your own resentment will infect the very quality of *your* life. This makes for a long and difficult journey.

Several *survivors who have become caregiver* to a spouse diagnosed with an illness have shared that it was easier as the survivor. How could this be? Survivors who become caregivers cite the tremendous helplessness of their new role. For example, the survivor knows just how much pain he or she is in, but the caregiver is left to speculate, never really knowing. And it's not just survivors turned caregivers who believe it's more difficult as caregiver. Many survivors whose partners never get ill think being the survivor is easier.

Whether or not it's easier as survivor or caregiver is subjective. But here's some hard science. A recent study in *Age and Aging* found that the increased burden experienced by someone caring for an ill loved one was significantly related to worsening health for that caregiver. And over 50 percent of the caregivers in the study showed measurable signs of depression.[11] Caregivers, your health is your responsibility. Please honor it.

Chapter Fifteen

Road Weary: Exploring Emotional Fatigue for Survivors, Caregivers, and Medical Professionals

*I*f you have ever driven cross-country, you know how desperately at times you may want to pull off the highway to rest. This "I'm done" feeling often comes with the landscape of illness, especially when treatment protocols are long and repeated. This "I'm done" feeling for the survivor might come in not wanting to see another needle, or in just wanting to stop it all. For caregivers, the "I'm done" exhaustion might hit in the middle of the night as memories flash of the survivor in pain. The "I'm done" feeling in medical professionals can register mid-shift with the thought, "I can't talk to one more patient tonight." All these "I'm done" experiences could be signs of emotional fatigue: road weariness.

Emotional fatigue, as described below, is not the same as burnout. Here are the principle differences between burnout and emotional fatigue.

• *Burnout comes from ongoing dissatisfaction,* which may be the product of, for example, repeated hassles with an insurance company, or lack of staff. *Emotional fatigue is born of trauma,* like hearing that you or the person you love has a life-threatening illness, or repeatedly telling others this news.

• *Burnout is usually slow to build and slow to dissipate,* like the mounting frustration with an insurance company, or staff shortages, and the slow recession of these frustrations once there is resolution. *Emotional fatigue comes on very quickly and intensely and usually leaves with similar speed,* like the days you can't sleep because you keep reliving the instant you heard the words, "You have sclera derma," or the instant you, a nurse, told those words to a twenty-six-year-old newlywed.

• *Thoughts related to burnout* may be persistent, like, "This insurance company is making me crazy," or, "I just can't keep covering these shifts." However, they *generally are not intrusive,* meaning they don't stop you in your tracks.

• *Thoughts related to emotional fatigue, on the other hand, can feel like stabs in the heart, and are intrusive.* They have the power to break concentration, rest, and conversations. These intrusive thoughts are often accompanied by images. For example, the survivor may have a flash of seeing him or herself in distress after a surgery. Or, the caregiver may have to turn from the computer at work to collect composure, struck by an image of the survivor wrestling with terror. A medical professional may almost have an accident driving home, distracted by haunting images of a young mother crying out with anger from the news of a recurrence.

• *People feeling burnout usually commiserate.* Couples dealing with a diagnosis may talk at dinner about the insurance problem. Nurses may walk to lunch discussing the short staff situation.

People feeling emotional fatigue often keep their

startling images and thoughts to themselves: "This is my husband with Alzheimer's, and he doesn't need my fear," or "This is my job. I'm supposed to be strong and available." Consequently, those dealing with emotional fatigue feel isolated and often withdraw, cutting themselves off from life-giving support.

Emotional fatigue and compassion fatigue are close cousins. For more information about the signs and symptoms of compassion fatigue, check out Charles R. Figley's book, *Compassion Fatigue: Secondary Traumatic Stress Disorders from Treating the Traumatized.*[12]

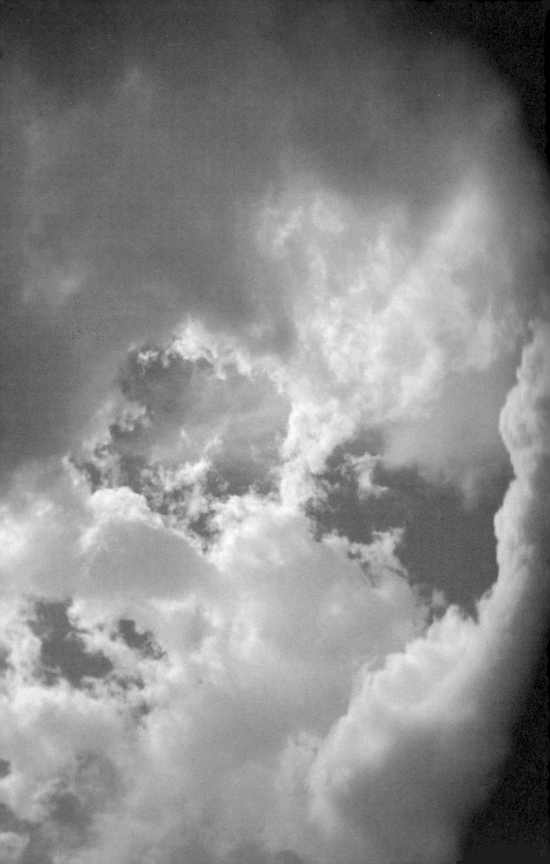

Chapter Sixteen

Rest Stop #5: Clearing the Clouds of Trauma and Anxiety for All Involved

During the journey beyond diagnosis, painful and traumatic moments are often revisited by the survivor, the caregiver, and the medical professional. When this happens, anxiety and fear usually come along. As one survivor said, "It's not fear I feel. It's terror." Anxiety, even when not accompanied by traumatic images, is one of the most frequently experienced emotions on the disease journey. Anxiety, like depression, is something most of us have learned to avoid or push away. Pushing anxiety or traumatic images away seems to give them power. These difficult experiences may intensify when "pushed against." An alternative means for relieving the pressure of anxiety and traumatic images is offered through the following exercise. Of course, if your traumatic images or heightened anxiety persist, consult a professional.

Clearing the Clouds of Trauma and Anxiety

Step 1. See your experience as a distant cloud
Step 2. Notice the cloud coming, passing through, and going
Step 3. Notice the light between the clouds

Step 1. See Your Experience as a Distant Cloud

Anyone who has dealt with recurring traumatic

images or anxiety knows they tend to cloud you. They can make thoughts foggy and difficult. Concentration becomes less and less possible.

Frank Herbert in his book *Dune* shares some valuable notions about anxiety. His basic message is that you are not your fear. You may see its coming and its going, but you are not your fear.[13] What a profound concept. When full with traumatic images or anxiety, you may feel like the self is lost and there is nothing else but the painful pictures or the fear. This "narrowed vision" compounds the anxiety, and fear expands exponentially.

In a previous chapter, we spoke about the natural startle response and its impact on the body's chemistry. Anxiety can create the same physical change. The difference, however, is that while the startle response is usually triggered by an external event, anxiety may often be induced by a seed thought or image from inside you. This scary, initial seed thought generates a second fearful thought, then another, and you're off to the races. The mind then feels like it's whirling. Eventually, the nervous system reacts to this internally generated feeling of fear like it does the startle response, cutting oxygen to the brain and sending it to the limbs. Thinking then becomes difficult. The brain is lacking the fuel it needs to do its job. Soon, there is nothing but feelings—dark, scary feelings.

By taking Step 1 of this exercise, **seeing your experience as a distant cloud,** you are stepping slightly out of your difficult feelings that have been set off by a scary thought. In using the cloud image, the mind gains an instant of objectivity from the fearful thoughts and feelings. The objectivity engages the brain in a slightly different way, and the body reacts by feeding the brain a little more oxygen. This begins to reverse, if only slightly, the downward spiral of anxiety, creating a chance to initiate a shift into a place of more peace.

What does it mean to see your **experience as a distant cloud?** It's a simple visualization. First of all, imagine that you are in a stadium or theatre. See yourself sitting high away from the field or stage. Next, imagine the traumatic incident that you keep flashing back to taking place on the field or stage, far away from you. Maybe your trauma is related to seeing yourself or the one you love in pain after another surgery. See that "scene" happening on the distant field or stage. Or if you are managing anxiety, visualize your fear "out there" away from you. Just watch this scene for a moment, without feeling, as if it belonged to someone else—like a scene from a play.

It's most important to *witness* your experience in this distant way. Stay with this part of Step 1 until you have the sense that your experience is *down there* on the field, or *out there* on the stage. Be patient and try not to wrestle with the visualization.

Once you see in the mind's eye your experience as distant from you, imagine that all the feelings associated with this scene gently rise up above the scene in the form of a cloud that is still "out there." Next, manipulate this cloud of feelings. Make the cloud go farther away from you. Make the cloud go back down to the scene. Have the cloud rise high, then left and right, still at a distance. Realize the mastery you have with this cloud containing your feelings.

As you stay with the cloud image, you are inviting your body, at the parasympathetic level, to begin to return to a less fearful state. You are calling your awareness out of your feelings and into an objective mind, by working with the image. In this way, you redial your chemistry. You will likely notice that it becomes easier to hold the image of the cloud because your body is beginning to send even more oxygen to your brain.

Step 2. Notice the Cloud Coming, Passing Through,
and Going

The cloud coming: When you're ready, invite the cloud containing your difficult feelings to rise up, still at a distance, to your eye level. Hold the cloud there, at eye level, a comfortable distance from you. At this point, the cloud and your feelings are still "out there."

Now, at your command, have the cloud of feelings begin to approach you from the front. Take this at your own pace. As the cloud of your feelings begins to approach, allow yourself to feel the difficult emotions the cloud contains, but only slightly, with the cloud still away from you, but coming closer.

Use your mastery with the cloud to manage how close you let the cloud of feelings come. The closer the cloud gets, the more you feel those difficult emotions. The farther away the cloud, the less you feel the feelings contained there.

Now, see yourself as a huge window screen, with great big holes between the wires of the screen.

Next, invite the cloud of your difficult emotions to come closer, and as it does, notice that the difficult feelings contained in the cloud are more intensely felt. You're in charge of the cloud. If the feelings get too intense, have the cloud back away. See a big fan blowing it away if you need to. Stay in charge of the cloud as best you can.

The cloud passing through: At your beckoning, have the cloud make contact with you, as the huge window screen, and notice the cloud beginning to pass through you. As it does, the difficult feelings contained there will feel more and more intense, until the emotions reach their most intense level as you—the screen—are full with the cloud.

Now the cloud is passing through. At this point, you will feel your most difficult emotions held in the cloud. Have the cloud continue to pass through you as a screen. If you want the cloud and its emotions to move through you more quickly, use the big fan again. Or, imagine someone or something behind you, pulling the cloud through and out of you. Let your mind create whatever image it needs to manage the cloud of difficult emotions in the way that helps you the most. As a screen, you can open the spaces between your wires, allowing the cloud to move through you more freely.

Noticing the *passing through* of the cloud is the toughest part. It means standing in the presence of your difficult emotions, full on. But keep some part of you outside the emotions, as an objective witness to it all—the part that created the stadium or theatre scene. It's like watching a movie, but the movie is you.

Now, apply these first two steps to the experience of anxiety. First, you imagine that your anxiety can be seen in the form of a cloud. Visualizing your anxiety in this way, you might say to yourself, "Yes, here comes the cloud of my anxiety. I notice that my mind is just starting to speed up." Or you might notice your stomach beginning to feel funny, or your heart beating a bit faster. This is noticing the front edge of your cloud: the coming. At this point, many folks do things to *not feel* the full thrust of the cloud. They get busy, or overreact with someone, or have someone else talk about their feeling, so as not to feel the fear anymore.

Now is the perfect opportunity to go through your anxiety instead of around it. When you go through it, it is less likely to keep chasing you. This is the art. This is the place you begin to create the possibility of less anxiety in your life. As strange as it may seem, this is where you initiate a shift into more peace. Oddly enough, it requires doing the very opposite of what you may be inclined to do. Rather than dodging or escaping the fear, this exercise invites you to move into it.

Acknowledge "the cloud" of approaching anxiety, stay with that image, and notice the cloud is getting closer and the anxiety is getting more intense. Breathe. Let the cloud of fear, with your full awareness and focus on its very intensity, pass through you, as a screen.

Remember, you are not your fear. The rest of you is still alive and vital. You are simply being visited at this moment, this period, by this cloud of fear. Stay with it. Let it *move through you.* Stop and let the fear do the moving. It too, shall pass.

Noticing fear passing through takes much courage, but the power you will develop as a person by this practice will be worth having. By noticing the anxiety, with all its fury, pass through, you essentially begin to reclaim the power that the cloud—the anxiety—contains. That power belongs to you.

Noticing the cloud of anxiety *passing through* might sound like: "Oh, I'm no longer on the edges of this cloud of anxiety. I'm right in the middle of it now. My fear is really strong. I'm feeling very scared. It's dark in here. I don't like this feeling at all. It feels like the fear is bigger than I am. Man. I know I'm in the worst part right now."

The cloud going: You did it. You noticed your trauma and/or your anxiety *coming* and *passing through* you. Keep noticing. Notice that the cloud is thinning out because it has moved almost completely through you, the screen. The cloud is *going:* "OK, I don't feel quite as uncomfortable or anxious as I did a few minutes ago. I'm still somewhat uncomfortable, but I think it's better." Keeping the image alive like this keeps you mindful. The mindfulness helps keep more blood/oxygen in your brain. That breaks the grip of the anxiety.

Now see the cloud fully behind and away from you, and take note of the difference in the intensity of your emotions. The farther the cloud gets from you, the less you feel the difficult emotions contained there, and the more comfortable you become.

Notice that the sense of trauma or anxiety may not be as severe as it was when you started the exercise: "Oh, you know what, I don't feel as scared as I did twenty minutes ago." By noticing this change, you begin to give your difficult emotions a form. Every form has a beginning, a middle, and an end. By working with your traumatic experience or anxiety in this way, you give it a form. It then no longer seems omnipresent, unruly, all-powerful, and unending. Rather, your fear will become just your fear. Many who have tried this process report a sense of relief in feeling separate from their fear. It is still their fear, but the "separateness" seems to rob fear of some of its power.

With time and practice, you will likely notice that the clouds come and go a little quicker. Then you might notice that the clouds come less often. Be patient.

Changing your internal landscape like this may take some time.

Step 3. *Notice the Light Between the Clouds*

The more you **notice the light between the clouds**, the more power you give the light. What the heck does that mean? The first two steps of this technique have encouraged you to give your difficult emotions full attention, *when they are present*. This last step promotes the idea that it is equally important to give full attention to what's present when your fear isn't: the peace, the absence of difficult emotions, the *light between the clouds*.

Between every cloud, there is light. Most people prefer light to darkness. However, when regularly dealing with difficult emotions, some forget to notice the light. In an anxious, uncomfortable emotional state, it is possible to overlook the absolute knowledge that there are periods, however brief, when the clouds part, the difficult emotions wane, and light is visible. There's a second of clarity or peace or trust.

Anxiety and peace, darkness and light, cloudy and clear—these are all simply states of mind. They are not enemies or allies. When one state is seen as good, the other is automatically established as evil or wrong or unhealthy. The task then becomes overcoming the enemy. Anxiety is a slippery enemy though. It feeds on attempts to overpower it. Fighting it tends to give it power. On the other hand, *just noticing fear* in an unattached, non-reactive way drains it of power, and then you feel better.

In the same way, when you notice that your mind is calm or peaceful or trusting, *that peaceful state* gains power. When you give full attention to the fact that you

are not having difficult emotions right now, the pleasant-
ness expands. So *noticing the light between the clouds*
becomes a sort of anxiety prevention.

A Next Step Approach

*Having learned to allow the difficult feelings to move
through you* by noticing the clouds and the light, you
may be ready for another discipline. Let me give you an
example. Say you are two years post-treatment for
mesothelioma and about to have another semi-annual
check up. Your post-treatment results have always been
positive, but most check-ups still raise your anxiety. You
find yourself thinking about a pain you felt a couple of
weeks ago, questioning, "Was that cancer?" Or maybe you
see yourself getting infused again and the anxiety builds.
Just after you were diagnosed, this anxiety before check-
ups was impossible. But you've practiced noticing the
coming, passing through, and going of your fear.
Consequently, the fear this time is not as intense.
Excellent. With the skill developed through working with
your own traumatic images or anxiety in this way, you
may be prepared for an additional approach.

As soon as your thoughts begin to induce fear before
your check-up, notice them as you did above, and then
transform them. You can do this by comfortably imagin-
ing that the fearful thoughts are infused with light, love,
peace, comfort, or all of the above. Take a breath. See the
fearful thoughts filling with light or love. Let this transformation visualization unfold naturally and comfortably.
As this transformation happens, gently introduce
thoughts based on your true experience: "I always feel
some anxiety at this time, but I always have good results.

I am going to let these inaccurate thoughts blend with my peace." In this way, you may transform the anxiety.

When first learning to work with your anxiety, this transformation visualization may be more difficult. Or, it might work well for you right from the start. Experiment. Use what works. With practice, the transformation approach may give you the power to shift your anxiety quickly. It's a curious process and feeling. Strong, clear, disciplined, and accurate thoughts can transform the anxiety when blended with compassion or hope. At times, there may be a sensation of internal fortification that you can almost sense, followed by the soft edges of peace and relaxation.

The big picture—**Clearing the Clouds of Trauma and Anxiety**—entails moving through the difficult emotions, rather than around. It is transforming rather than resisting. It means knowing that it is possible to have fear, yet choosing not to be afraid.

Cherish the light. Your anxiety is not you. You are so much more.

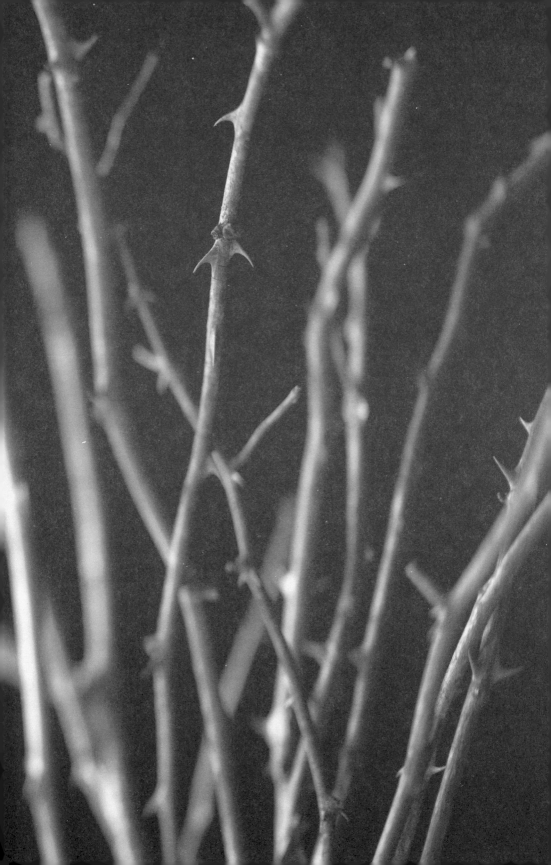

Chapter Seventeen

Potholes: Unexpected Emotions that Jar You

There comes a time in most long trips when you get sleepy. Things get a little blurry, you're in kind of an altered state, stripes on the highway have a hypnotic effect, and your head starts to bob. Hopefully, you either pull off the highway and rest, or something snaps you out of your sleepiness. This chapter deals with being snapped out of your quiet.

The white lines of the illness journey are the routines established through ongoing treatments and follow-up. Eventually, what was curious and engaging becomes standard fare, regardless of your role in the journey. Dialysis, blood draws, and physical therapy are just procedures. Blue radiation marks on your body are a bit old hat. You have become somewhat mesmerized by it all.

Treatment has worked; you're back to a regular job schedule; the family has adjusted to the "new" survivor; survivor and caregiver are looking and acting more like their old selves; and some of the pleasures of life are coming out of hibernation.

Early times of the journey had you awake and alert, either as the survivor, the caregiver, or the newly trained medical professional—so much to do and to learn. Any potholes on your road were skillfully avoided. Eyes were wide open then, and you noticed most everything. However, now that you've been on the highway awhile, you're lulled into a bit of a trance. It's when you are in this mental and emotional state of relative relaxation that you might hit a pothole.

For some, the jolt comes in the form of a glance. It's the sideways and unexpected glimpse of your scar or the scar of the person you love. Just like that, you're bowled over by a wave of emotions, thoughts, and internal experiences. Where is all this feeling coming from? The sight of your own body or your loved one's body has triggered a domino of reactions you were not ready for. All the old fears seem as strong as ever. Or maybe a wave of anger comes on. Maybe it's sadness— sadness that you, your body, your loved one's body, your spirit, and your family had to go through so much. And just like that, you are unmistakably back on the highway of the journey beyond diagnosis.

Kevin had a large tumor removed from a nasal passage. Immediately after surgery, his speech and appearance were both effected. He got through those times thankful to be alive and aware that corrective and plastic surgery would return most of his speech and appearance. They did. The post-surgery facial scar was strong, but Kevin was patient as the scar healed and became less visible. In group, he shared, "I'm glad to be here, to be breathing like you do, and looking forward to the rest of my life. This disease, odd as it may seem, has been a gift to me. My wife and I got closer through it. This scar is the least of my worries."

Months went by. Kevin spoke in group about family stuff, job issues, and what he was doing to take care of himself. Every once in a while, he would refer to his scar: "I'm fine with this. How I look is not a big deal."

And then one day Kevin came to group with a different message. "My wife and I had a portrait taken," he explained. "Big deal, right? Well, when the proofs showed up this week, something really hit me."

After a long pause, someone in the group asked, "What happened, Kevin?"

"It's hard to talk about. And I'm not exactly sure. All I know was when I saw myself in those pictures, something broke in me. My wife had to pull the pictures away, cause I was so mad. I could have ripped 'em up right there."

It took time in a couple of sessions for Kevin to discover what had happened. Early on, his anger was too powerful to be acknowledged. Some part of him knew that. Early on, Kevin developed other tools for getting through all that was being asked of him. This is a variety of the *emotional efficiency* discussed in a previous chapter. But now that the rest of his life was getting back to normal, Kevin had the strength to look into the face of his anger. The anger was strong, but so was Kevin, and eventually he got beyond even his intense anger. Seeing himself in those portraits was a pothole for Kevin.

A similar emotional "busting open" can be created by the pothole of waiting for test results. You were cruising along at a pretty good clip, you thought. The pothole, however, was lying there about two days out from getting that annual test result back, and it hit you as a powerful wave of fear. Once again, you find yourself on the road to recovery that you had nearly forgotten you were on.

One final circumstance that may be a pothole for some: everyone else's perfect life. This pothole has an odd shape. You're happy. So, too, are those you love. Then one day, pop—you're combing through a pile of emotions that sound like this: "My life isn't the same. I'm not the same. I didn't ask for this. All these people on TV, all my neighbors, so many of my family, they don't have a care in the world. But I have this emotional scar that illness caused." This hidden resentment is a pothole.

Potholes can show up years after treatment is successfully completed. And obviously, not everybody hits these potholes. Yet even the folks who travel forward from illness with glad hearts can hit sharp pockets of feelings they don't or can't predict. Knowing that potholes are out there may make your journey beyond diagnosis a little safer.

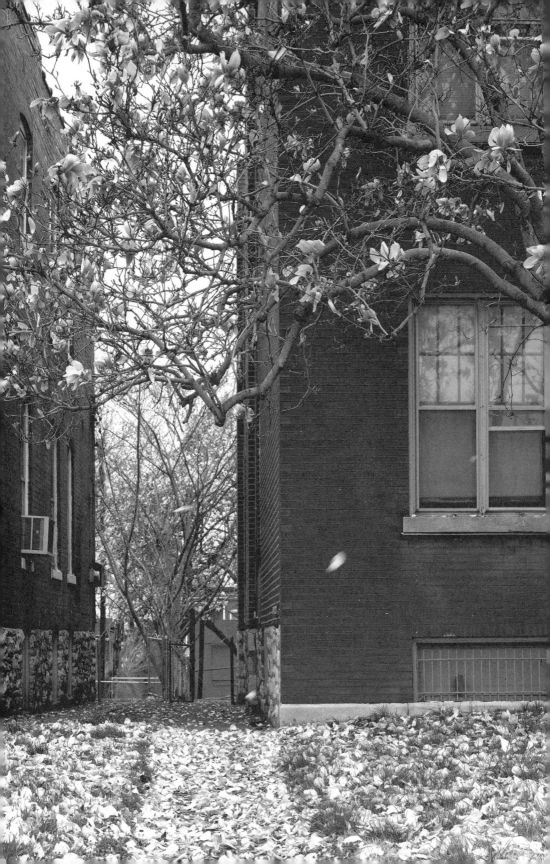

Chapter Eighteen

Rest Stop #6: A Quick Release Anxiety Tool–I Am More Than My Fear

Potholes on your journey beyond diagnosis often come with rapid onset anxiety. It might be the rush of panic just before test results or the racing mind when you, the one you love, or the person you treat finds a new pain or bump. Time on the journey makes these difficult moments more bearable, as experience teaches you the usefulness of gently being less reactive. But fear is powerful. The following exercise is offered as a tool to help rapidly release you from fear.

"I Am More Than My Fear"

Step 1. State what you observe
Step 2. Declare, "I am more than my fear"
Step 3. Breathe life into the rest of you

Step 1. State What You Observe

Each person has Stress Activated Signals (SAS) that indicate the onset of anxiety. When used effectively, these signals can help you manage that fear. First, identify your specific mental and physical SAS—those cues that tell you anxiety may be starting. Try to identify the one SAS that shows up earliest. Perhaps when you first become anxious, your mind starts to race or your heart beats faster. For some, the SAS may be sweaty palms or hot ears.

Once you know what your first SAS is, let it inform you that anxiety is beginning. Watch for it. As soon as you recognize this cue in yourself, **state what you observe.** For example, say to yourself, "Oh, my throat's getting dry. I can feel that. I know then that I'm beginning to get anxious." This simple act of thinking helps to physiologically interrupt the fear-based fight or flight reaction in your body.

Step 2. Declare, "I Am More Than My Fear"

Once you have observed the early signs of anxiety in yourself, declare, **"I am more than my fear."** Say it out loud if you want. With this declaration, you are creating within yourself the opportunity for something other than fear. Any time you *observe* your fear in such a way, you step outside that fear. In doing so, you make contact with the rest of who you are in that very same moment. That fear then becomes only a fraction of the total self. Plus, the words spoken in this step support the idea that your fear is always and only a *part* of you.

Step 3. Breathe Life into the Rest of You

So there you are: your fear, and the rest of you. Leave the fear be. Notice it, but don't try to make it go away by pushing against it. It will push back, and you could get stuck in the struggle. Instead, **breathe life into the rest of you.** Take a deep breath, and imagine your breath traveling to an aspect of yourself that you wish to expand, or feel more fully. Maybe you want to feel more trusting. So, as you inhale, see your breath going to, expanding, and giving life to the trust you know exists inside you. You know this because you've felt trust before. Breathe life into your trust.

Perhaps you want to breathe life into more than your trust. So be it. See that happening. The number of qualities, feelings, or attributes you can expand far out number the fear. Fear isn't bad. It's just a small and sometimes powerful part of the total you. As a matter of fact, Joseph Hiller claims, "Fear is excitement without breath."

So, breathe life into as much of the rest of you as you like. See the breath going to all those other aspects of you, making them open or grow. If you like, see the rest of you dancing as you breathe life into it. *Notice* the fear, and invite the rest of you to shine.

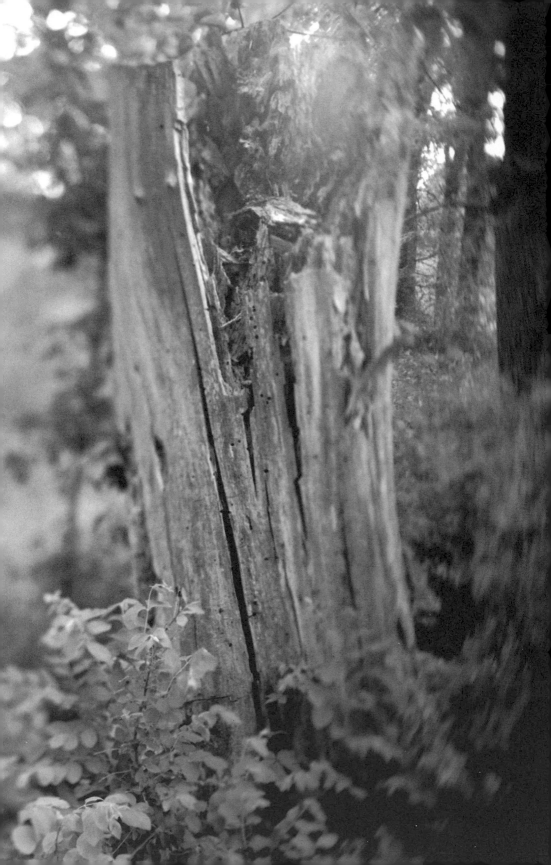

Chapter Nineteen

Crashes: Major Interruptions in Your Recovery Journey

With plenty of time spent on the highway, a crash is unfortunately possible. A crash is an unexpected and sometimes emotionally expensive interruption in your trip. This chapter presents some of the major sources of mental, emotional, relational, and even spiritual crashes for those on the journey beyond diagnosis. The later part of the chapter explores how strong emotion may be responded to, in general.

Recurrence/Relapse

The number one cause of crashes on the illness journey is **recurrence/relapse**. The emotional, mental, relational, and even spiritual damage caused by recurrence/relapse can be severe for all involved. For the survivor, feeling emotionally whole after a recurrence/ relapse can be difficult. Survivors—and others involved—may be painfully cut by the words, "The disease has come back." Who wouldn't be?

Hope seems to be the biggest piece in this puzzle. It's hard to recover hope with a second occurrence of an illness. For many who experience illness recurrence/ relapse, hope does not recur as sure or as fast or as strong: "The more you hope, the harder you fall." The same fear of hoping may strike the caregiver or invade the medical professional's spirit.

Some find mustering the strength to go forward very difficult. Imagine finishing a grueling marathon, one that drained life from every aspect of you, and sitting to rest, when someone runs over yelling, "What are you doing? That really wasn't the finish line. This is an ultramarathon. You have ten more miles to go. Get up. Get running." There's a lot you might like to do right then; standing up and running is not one of them. It makes sense that a recurrence/relapse can cause real emotional trauma.

If you or the person you love is responding to recurrence/relapse, please be patient. There is a level of emotional fragility that is extremely difficult for anyone other than someone else who has dealt with recurrence/relapse to truly comprehend. Dreams just rebuilt are now dashed. Of course, they can be built again, but if the dreams were yours, recurrence/relapse can make them very, very hard to envision.

Relationships may be contorted at this time. The survivor feels like anything but a survivor. It's easier at the time of recurrence/relapse to feel victimized. When that happens, many tough questions can arise: "Will I have the strength to keep fighting?" "Do I want to fight?" "Will fighting make a difference?" "Am I better off to end treatment and go for quality in the life I have left?" "Where is God?" "Should I keep loving my children, or is it best to start distancing from them?" "What's the point of all this?" "Can I endure?" The caregiver is asking many of these same questions.

Try not to let the questions scare you. Give yourself permission to feel whatever you feel and hold on to whatever gives you strength, if that's what you decide you want. If you can, allow whatever emotions appear to pass through you like clouds. They may be powerfully intense, but they are still only feelings. The rest of you is still there.

End of Treatment

Yes, even when the prognosis is positive, the successful **end of treatment** has thrown survivors (and sometimes caregivers) off course. Survivors report that an unusual fear can come over them as they walk from the doctor's office after a final treatment. This fear may be confusing. The end of treatment is a time when those around the survivor applaud. Generally, everybody's pretty up. Fear in the survivor at this point can be met with the question, "How can you feel bad at a time like this?" No safety net.

Treatment has been the survivor's ally—the lifeline, as one survivor described it. Treatment is the one thing that kept hope alive. Treatment was a concrete, measurable way to know the illness was being overcome. Without treatment, many survivors feel there's no one minding the store. The rush of unexpected emotions when treatment ends is enough to crash some survivors.

Emotional Unpacking

There is one more major cause of crashes, and this one seems especially perplexing: **emotional unpacking**. Earlier, we spoke of *emotional packing*—putting all the emotions that can come with a diagnosis away, so full attention may be given to the matters of treatment, surgery, and procedures. But what is packed must be unpacked. When and how the unpacking happens can be unsettling.

There was a woman—Joan—who joined a group nearly eight months after her treatment was over. Joan's prognosis was excellent. Everything in her life was returning to normal: "Mom, are you going to take me to practice?" and, "Honey, we're going to dinner with Bob and Cindy Friday night, OK?" Not OK. For some reason, nothing really felt OK to Joan. Not long after joining the group, Joan made contact with her disappointment. At first she couldn't figure it out. Then it started to get clear.

Joan felt that everybody wanted everything to be just like it used to be. At some level, so did Joan. But at another level, she knew it would never be and she was disappointed at people pressing her to be the mother, wife, friend, and person she no longer was.

Joan felt that family and friends wanted to act like nothing ever happened. Joan knew she couldn't be the same person she used to be; she didn't want to. Too much had impacted her body, mind, and spirit. And Joan resented the fact that people started giving her the "get over it" message: "Look, I know it was hard on you, but your treatment was over a long time ago, and you're fine. Thank God. Let's put it behind us."

But now Joan was beginning to feel the emotions she had packed away early on, like fear and sadness and anger. The last thing she felt she could do was put it all behind her. In group, she was opening what felt to her like a whole suitcase full of tough emotions.

Sound familiar? It was Joan's time to unpack. Joan did great through the initial throes of diagnosis and treatment. She got back on her horse and started to ride. Then it hit. All the feelings that had been packed in the beginning of her journey beyond diagnosis were now busting out, begging to be unpacked, and a few other feelings had been added along the way. This unpacking may not happen until many months, and even years, after successful treatment.

And the survivor isn't the only one completely taken off guard by this unpacking process. Everybody in the family is baffled by the survivor's emotionality at this time. Understanding comes in handy here. And sometimes it's the survivor who wants to act like nothing ever happened, leaving the caregiver in a quandary.

Emotional Efficiency

Joan, early in her trip, had unconsciously practiced **emotional efficiency**. Some part of her knew that venturing deep into all the feelings generated by diagnosis, surgery, and treatment was more than she could handle right then. Her whole self chose to pack the emotional stuff away to be unpacked later. *Later* usually becomes a time when things are better and settling down for the survivor. It's as if the whole person knows when it's safe to take this unpacking task on.

Here's another version of emotional efficiency. Sean was struggling to finish his treatment. Pain and fatigue were significant. In addition, Sean had just made it through a nasty divorce and his ex-wife was not helping. On top of that, his young daughter was developmentally disabled. When Sean started the group, he came with rage wrapped in lots of anxiety. His greatest anxiety was about dying and opening the door for his ex to gain custody of their child. For months he used the group to download his anxiety and anger. Then one week Sean seemed different. There was an air of peace about him.

The group asked Sean about his change: "I can't afford to be anxious any more." He went on to explain that when really anxious and angry, his pain got out of control, and when that happened, he couldn't feel any joy with his daughter. That simple awareness changed his life. Anxiety and anger registered now as wasteful. He had developed another sort of *emotional efficiency.*

Internal Accountant

With emotional efficiency and emotional unpacking, it's like there is some sort of inner accounting going on—as if an **internal accountant** has assumed responsibility for resource allocation. Early in the diagnosis experience, this accountant allocates internal resources for the most important matters: finding the right doctor, having surgery, healing the body, getting treatments. The accountant knows that in the beginning internal resources are being spent quickly and that revenues (experiences that greatly relieve stress or recharge the emotions) are minimal. Consequently, the precious internal resources are kept in reserve and only allocated to the most essential of needs.

At the start of the journey beyond diagnosis, emotional wellness is usually less vital than the need to control pain, heal wounds, or stop the illness. Consequently, little reserve is spent on emotions and they get put in an internal safe deposit box. This is usually good business on the part of the internal accountant. It is *emotionally efficient.*

Now once pain, illness, healing, etc. are addressed, the internal resources get replenished. With things returning to normal, joy is experienced, hope is recovered, relationships bring salve to the wounded heart and body, and everything begins to heal. This is all income for the internal accountant. The bank account inside is recovering.

And eventually, there are some extra internal resources to spend.

At this point, the internal accountant addresses the next order of business: paying off those emotional debts. There is no way to predict when this payoff is going to be rendered. Everybody's internal account gets depleted and recovers in different degrees, different ways, and at different times. Some survivors might address their deeper emotions while still in treatment. Other survivors contend with these emotions months after treatment stops. For some, paying down the emotional debt happens years later.

Nonetheless, the internal accountant is quite good at the job, and these emotional accounts will be paid off. If the internal accountant doesn't address these emotional debts, you might incur penalties.

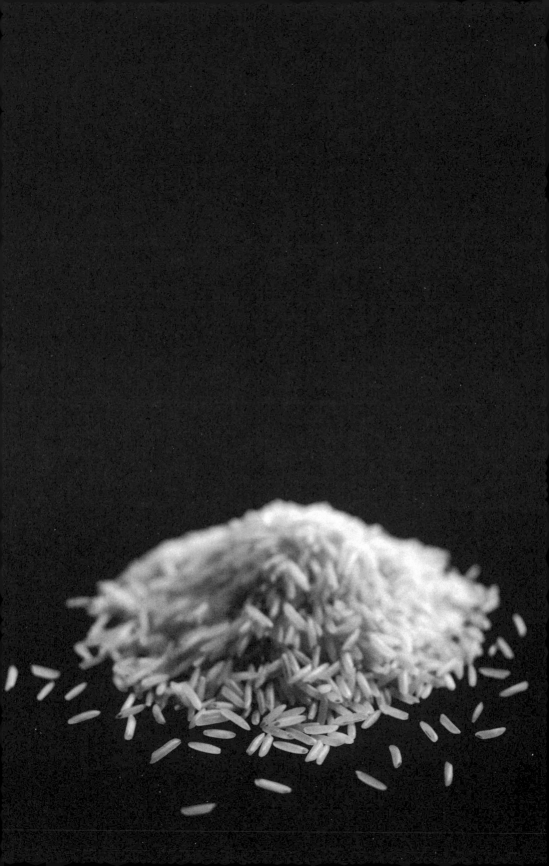

Chapter Twenty

Rest Stop #7: Feeding the Hungry Ghost–An Exercise for Responding to Depression

A "crash" as discussed in the previous chapter is a bout with depression. And in our culture, depression is generally considered something to avoid: an enemy. Yes, depression is difficult. Yes, serious and chronic depression may require professional support and even medication. But what would happen if you thought of depression as a messenger of sorts? What would change if you pushed less against this experience and instead made some room for it? This chapter describes an exercise based on such an approach to depression.

Make no mistake about it. Some feel their depression is the worst pain they have ever experienced. But when absolutely resisted, these troubling undulations of spirit become more than pain. When emotional pain is completely resisted, it gains power. With power, pain expands into suffering.

Unfortunately, there is little training for responding to tough feelings like sadness, fear, hurt, hopelessness, and anger. Consequently, these emotions often underpin depression. This discussion, this exercise, and this book are all offered to help you learn to acknowledge your tough feelings sooner, so as to mitigate depression.

This exercise is also presented to begin to shift your perception of depression from *enemy* to *informant*. An informant often appears as the enemy but eventually shares useful information.

When perceived as an enemy, depression becomes the

object of appeasement. People who see depression as the enemy act in ways designed to keep this difficult emotion at bay. These people were probably taught this pattern by important adults in their young lives who themselves never learned how to respond to tough feelings. Pushing depression away is part of our culture. But unfortunately, the one who appeases the crocodile, as Winston Churchill put it, is simply the last one eaten.[14]

So, how can you respond to depression besides appeasing it? What else can you do when you begin to experience that "blueness"; the feeling that things just aren't making you very happy? Here's the story of the Hungry Ghost to answer that question.

In Tibet, children are taught to carry a grain of rice in their pockets. The rice, children are told, should be thrown into the mouth of the Hungry Ghost, should it approach. The Hungry Ghost is depicted having rows and rows of razor sharp teeth in gaping jaws. So what good is a grain of rice? Legend has it that when you throw a single grain of rice into the fierce jaws of the Hungry Ghost, its mouth immediately closes, revealing a tiny body capable of consuming nothing more. The child's scary emotions of fear, sadness, and disappointment are represented by the monster and all its teeth.

In applying this story to adults with depression, the Tibetan wisdom is clear: when responding to difficult emotions, it helps to face them and then nurture them in some way. Only after acknowledging and nurturing these emotions can you discover what is true: the feelings feared are only a perceived monster. These poignant emotions only have the power they are given.

With this notion in mind, here are three steps for dealing with depression, especially in its early stages. People with serious or prolonged depression should consult a professional.

Feeding the Hungry Ghost—An Exercise for Responding to Depression

Step 1. Face your own discomfort
Step 2. Nourish it with your attention
Step 3. Listen for information

Step 1. Face Your Own Discomfort

To do this, you usually have to slow down enough to make contact with your discomfort. And just like the Tibetan child who is invited to look into the jaws of the Hungry Ghost, looking into the eyes of your own pain may be very scary.

Slowing down will likely mean doing less of the things you've done to keep the pain at bay. Maybe that means exercising less, or feeling *other* peoples' emotions less, or controlling another's behavior less, or spending less time in the office, or shopping less, or eating more, or any of the many other drugging actions that can numb emotional pain. Stopping these actions in yourself is a monumental task, especially if it's how you have managed the pain most of your life. The stronger your difficult emotions, the stronger your behaviors are likely to have been to numb those emotions.

Be patient with yourself. There's a reason you don't want to feel what's in you. As you slow down and begin to thaw, all that you have been anesthetizing yourself against will start to smart. You may need some counsel at this point. At the very least, it will help to talk to your mate or a close friend. Journaling is useful, too.

Step 2. Nourish It with Your Attention

All right, you've slowed things down—you're

facing your own discomfort. Now set an intention in your heart, mind, or spirit. You can do this through prayer, or meditation, or simple silence. In responding to depression, your intention might be to gain awareness of what is at the center of your pain. In a sense, you now seek to understand the depression by offering it your attention. Ask yourself over the next couple of weeks to simply notice your inner life. There's nothing to change or do at this point. If you make this process of attention "an assignment," you set yourself up to get an "A" or an "F," and that may cause more pain.

Instead, just notice. Invite the non-judgmental observer within yourself to simply witness what seems to be true. Like how often do you feel the depression and what, when, where, or how does it tend to get stronger? What core feelings live inside the depression: anger, sadness, hopelessness, hurt, disappointment, terror? How much territory do the feelings claim in your emotional landscape? Does that change? How old is the part of you that seems to be having the tough emotions? If you had to say, where do the feelings show up in your body: your head, your chest, your belly? Is this a place you have physical ailments? There are no right or wrong answers. There is no task to master. You just want to get to know this "blue" part of yourself a bit better. You are "nourishing" the depression with your attention.

Step 3. Listen for Information

Now that you've slowed down and nourished your depression by paying more attention to it, your depression might have a message for you. It may want to be an informant. Listen.

Deep within you there is a part that is very wise and understands more than you might believe. That wisdom is best heard when you still yourself and earnestly wait for understanding. *Wait* is the operant word here. Let the understanding come to you. This may take time. Your dreams might kick up as you slow down. They can teach about the depression, too.

In listening to your depression with that wisest part of who you are, you may discover that your depression is much older than your illness. In the quiet, you perhaps learn that when you were seven years old you were having pains in your gut just like the pain you feel now with your depression. Maybe that awareness reveals a very important connection between how you interacted with others then and how you interact with others now. As a result of this awareness, you may begin to interact *differently* in certain relationships now, and then your gut feels better.

Maybe you listen deeply and discover that you have not honored your own instincts about the best way to treat your illness. Consequently, at the next visit to your doctor, you discuss new treatment options that feel more true for you. Though it was difficult for you to speak with your doctor this way, the doctor surprises you by agreeing completely. A few days later, you notice that you feel less depressed.

Finally, through listening, perhaps you realize for the first time that you aren't *always* "blue." You're only blue after spending time with certain people. More listening reveals that those people find fault with you. Slowly, you see those people less, and your depression lifts.

Through practice of the three steps offered in this Rest Stop exercise, you will likely learn that the closer attention you pay to your emotional experience, including your depression, the more it can teach you. Respect it. It is not an enemy. It's an informant.

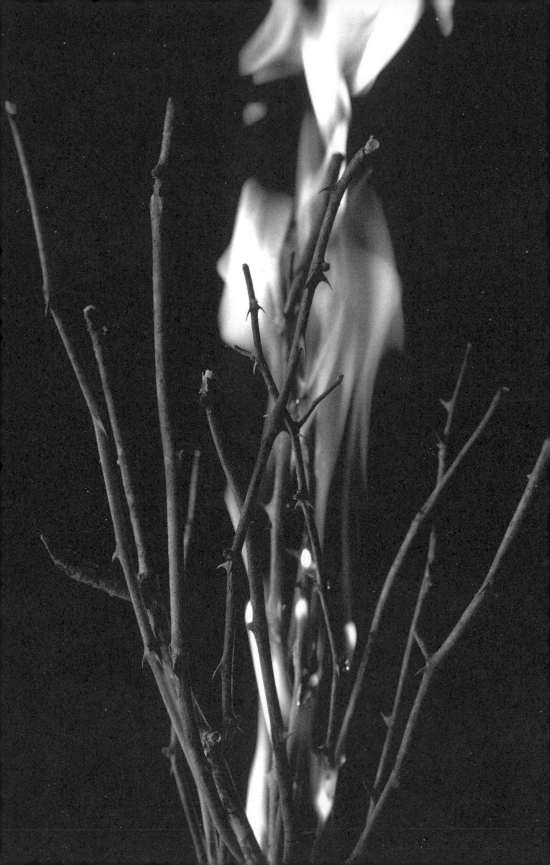

Chapter Twenty-One

Road Rage: Understanding Anger

Anybody who's been on the road long enough is bound to have a flare-up or two. You get uncomfortable away from home so long, you want to get off the road, you're tired, and you're on your last nerve. Everybody in the car knows it and probably feels much the same way. With enough detours and potholes and potential crashes during the journey beyond diagnosis, there could be some anger. The truth is, many people wrestle with this emotion—anger—whether or not they are ill. It seems to be an especially loaded emotion for most. Like the general population, many illness survivors have an "all or nothing" relationship with their own anger.

"I don't even know what anger feels like," Francie reflected. "I get scared and sad and disappointed, but I don't get angry. I guess I don't know how to get angry," she admitted, sounding both sad and surprised at the same time. Francie was twenty-three when diagnosed with lung cancer. Her parents lived nearby, but the relationship with them was strained. And though she had some friends, Jack, her boyfriend, was her closest ally.

In the beginning, Jack stood by her. However, that relationship thinned. And five months into our work together, Francie found out that Jack was seeing someone else. While this loss was extremely painful, it provided Francie a way to befriend her anger.

"Francie, you've openly described how hurt you are by Jack," I began one session. "You've also told me nothing makes sense anymore. What other emotional or physical reactions have you noticed over the past week?"

"It's weird," she said, "that you ask about physical

reactions. I haven't had treatment for two weeks, but my stomach has been a wreck the last couple days."

"How is your stomach right now?" was my next question.

"Not good, why?"

"Well," I answered, "maybe your stomach has something to say to you."

With this as the introduction, Francie began a venture into her own anger. Unaware of what was happening internally, she kept a log of what was going on in her stomach, her mind, and her emotions. In the weeks that followed, Francie began to make connections that slowly surfaced hidden anger. First, she dug through bitter resentment at Jack. Under this anger, Francie found resentment about her physical situation and the illness. And then under that anger, Francie discovered a part of herself that was nearly rageful. This deeper, older anger, however, had little to do with her boyfriend or her illness. Through this process, Francie's emotional congestion was beginning to clear, and so was her spirit.

It's important to say, plain and simple, the best way to clear the congestion of any emotion is through it, not around it. Many suggest that anger is a bad emotion and should be avoided. But it's the very act of avoiding that creates congestion. Like any difficult emotion, when anger is acknowledged and accepted, new action rises up naturally. Working with anger, you learn of its guiding force, and you consequently create a life that is more comfortable. And in this new life, as we will see later in the chapter, you may find yourself feeling less and less anger, *genuinely*, and not from going around it but from going through it.

Understanding Anger

So, what's behind the widespread struggles with the emotion of anger? While responses to this question can be complex, I'd like to keep it simple. Your early life environment may have taught you to keep your anger to yourself. Consequently, your anger may have gotten stuck inside you.

Before we discuss how such emotional congestion may occur, it's important to talk about blame. There is none. Not of significant people in your past. Not of parents. Not of you. We all do and have done the best we can. Blame is of no good to anyone. This discussion of anger is about understanding. The heart carries the past. That past can be wonderful and filled with love, and that comes through in all the relationships you have today. Your past may also have involved other encounters and circumstances that left a wound on your heart—it's the human condition. That wound *also* comes through in all the relationships you have today.

However, our discussion here is about going forward. When you understand how wounds of the past influence experiences of the present, you position yourself to create a better future. This instinctive healing process flows naturally from understanding.

With that said, here's one way to understand how anger may be stuck inside an adult. Many experience anger as all or nothing because they saw it as all or nothing in the important people from their young lives. Couples often pair around this anger equation. One has outbursts of anger, and the other allows it. Another way to think of it is that one member of the pair tends toward aggression, and the other toward passivity. And these tendencies are not gender specific.

We generally feel more accepting of the passive behavior and judmental of the aggressive behavior. Truth is, both aggressive and passive behavior can be powerful. Aggressive power simply tends to be more apparent, direct, and abusive. Passive power tends to be more difficult to identify, less direct, and more manipulative. We often see agressive power as non-caring and passive power as caring. This may be inaccurate.

It goes without saying that anger at the level of rage is usually inappropriate, destructive and brings violence into relationships and homes. Yet is is also clear that passive power can be insidious and difficult to heal from. But most importantly, both the aggressive and passive responses to anger send a very clear message to the young child growing up in this environment: "Don't get angry or you'll get hurt."

Yes, anger is a powerful emotion and, even when appropriately expressed, can feel *overpowering* to the person receiving the anger. Consequently, the healthy expression of anger may appear to some as a display of power. And if the recipient of the anger feels he or she is being controlled by that anger, he or she may try to shut that anger down. This is the rub, and why healthy anger is sometimes thwarted. And healthy anger, when thwarted, may congest the individual. Suppressed and congested anger, as we discussed in Chapter 5, may compromise the immune function.

So how did this dynamic play out in the life of a child whose anger is stuck inside as an adult? The aggressive member of the pair in the young one's life may have been threatened by the child's anger. This may have been acted out in a way that scared or punished the child. Consequently, the child heard, literally or figuratively, "Don't you dare get angry with me!"–anger stuck inside. And the passive member, by allowing the anger of his or her spouse, also said to the young one, "Keep your anger to yourself, like I do"–anger stuck inside. This is in no way suggesting that children not be disciplined. It is suggesting that children have a right to likes and dislikes, and sometimes those get expressed through anger.

One final thought for understanding: People who are threatened by and therefore thwart the healthy anger of others are usually carrying a lot of hurt and fear beneath their own anger. These people probably had their own young anger thwarted. And people who passively allow the unhealthy anger of others probably witnessed that same allowance in an important relationship in their own lives. This is the anger cycle. In this cycle, there is a lot of fear. And when fear is present, love is not. Sadly, love is what everyone in the cycle wanted in the first place, and it is the one thing that can break the anger chain.

The Self, Saying No, and Congested Anger

Countless survivors have said they never *learned* to say no. Saying no is a way of being who you are. Saying no is one way the self emerges. Saying no is often born from a message inside the self that takes the external form of anger. When done appropriately, this expression of anger is very healthy and natural. Of course, it often just shows up in children, i.e., the terrible two's. It seems, though, many individuals and illness survivors were never allowed or *taught* to pay attention to their anger and say no; that is, their authentic self was given limited support.

Independent thinking, opinion expressing, and acknowledging one's own emotions are all ways the self emerges. "Baseball is boring," "I think the yellow shoes are prettier," "I don't like brussel sprouts," "You scared me," and "Stop tickling me," are all ways a child might give voice to the emerging self and say, "no." My sense is that these very expressions of self were discounted or ignored in the early lives of many who, as adults, struggle today with how to respond to their own anger. These are the seeds of congested anger.

Origins of congested, old anger take many forms. The source described here is a type of neglect just outlined. This is not neglect in the traditional sense—all the essentials like shelter, food, clothing, and even love may have been provided. Instead, the neglect described here is more likely an unconscious act of suppression by important people in the young person's life.

As the young emerging self with its anger was suppressed by significant others, and trained not to come out, the individual's anger and true self got stuck inside. There are two basic ways the stuck self, with its anger, manages this suppression: anger turned in against the self or anger regularly boiled over and turned out against others. These two approaches produce the compliant "say-yes" youth-adult who tends to agree with and support others, or the aggressive "impose-yes" youth-adult who tends to demand agreement and support *from* others. There is always a third option. That option here would be the youth-adult who may agree with and support others and expresses very little anger, then explodes, and demands.

It makes sense that more of the compliant say-yes adults tend to suffer illness than the impose-yes adults. After all, in the say-yes population, there was no apparent permission to send natural anger outside the self. So instead, the anger got turned in against the self, and as we established earlier, this can be very hard on the body.

Consequences of Unexpressed Anger

In many survivors, consistently unexpressed anger can turn back on the self in the form of shame, self-rejection, or poor esteem. A life of this produces "old anger." This old anger ferments, tears you up inside, and turns into resentment.

Adults who have not learned to say no, yet naturally desire mastery in their lives, often feel powerless. In response to that powerlessness, some attempt to hyper-control their surroundings. This could be the person who is extremely neat or extremely driven professionally. It might be the adult who tries to feel everyone else's feelings. It could be the adult whose humor comes at the expense of others. Or it might be the adult that pushes, criticizes, or overmanages, be it self, spouse, employee, or child.

Some who feel powerless attempt to feel mastery by having too much or too little food, too much or too little exercise, too much or too little sex, too much or too little structure, or too many techniques or substances to alter their mood. Unexpressed anger is not the only explanation for such behaviors, but it's often a piece of the puzzle. It bears repeating that this discussion is for understanding not blame. With understanding, you may be more able to accept yourself and others. When you bring compassion in, growth naturally follows. Life gets better. Who knew anger could be a doorway to fuller living?

On the other hand, life feels anything but full when people who never learned to say no find themselves in minimizing relationships as adults. How does this happen? These adults practice what they were taught: to say yes. That is, as children they learned it was safer, and they felt more valued when they agreed with the predominant opinion and kept their point of view to themselves. In the adult, this say-yes behavior attracts others who like to be said yes to. Consequently, the self that got stuck inside the child remains stuck in the adult. In extreme cases, these adults with a self stuck inside may find themselves in abusive situations. The result is more hurt and more fear.

Those who never learned to say no are often trained as children to be friendly and helpful and respectful. Friendliness, helpfulness, and respectfulness are good things. However, when you add those qualities to an adult who has never learned to say no, difficulties may arise. On the outside, these adults appear happy and are fun to be around. They can be generous with their time and money. And yet, these same folks often agree to more than they really want:

more work, more time, more donated money, more self-sac-
rificing. It's not uncommon for these people to work themselves sick and smile through it all. The adult is now repeating the childhood experience: the self is not being heard.
The resentment grows.

Life may not be easy for the impose-yes adult either.
Often, these frustrated individuals add layers to that pain by
their own actions, driving important people out of their
lives with anger. The impose-yes adult is then left without
the care and support that might heal their injuured hearts.

Whether turned in on the self, or out against others as
aggression or rage, the person who never learned to say no
travels with a lot of resentment. Louise Hay, an internation-
ally recognized self-help author and lecturer, was diagnosed
with cancer. Here is her take on illness and anger:

*I knew cancer was a disease of deep resentment that has
been held for a long time until it literally eats away at the body.
I had been refusing to be willing to dissolve all the anger and
resentment at "them" over my childhood. There was no time to
waste; I had a lot of work to do."*[15]

Befriending Your Anger

How does one make friends with anger? It starts by practicing the Triple A Exercise described in Chapter 6. By
acknowledging the anger, the fear, the hurt, and the pain,
you begin to invite the self to come out. This can be very
painstaking. Everything in you says, "Don't say it! Don't feel
it!" Acknowledging and expressing your anger—your self—
may have gotten you punished in some way as a little one.
Like a shy turtle, you'll keep withdrawing from this acknowledgment. That's OK. Stay with it. Take your time. By giving yourself time and patience, you are retraining yourself.
In this way, you begin to honor all of who you are, and self-
respect is given life. Once this happens, authenticity emerges.

As you grow in authenticity, you begin to notice what you like and what you don't like; what you feel and what you don't feel; what you want to do and what you don't want to do. The self is being breathed into. The self that was stuck inside is being born. How wonderful!

As you acknowledge and accept all that you are, you will act differently. People may not like that right away: "What happened to the person who was so easy to get along with, so friendly, and always said yes when you needed help?" Well, that person is still there. But now that person has opinions, with likes and dislikes. That person is taking better care of the self.

If you can, avoid the strong pull to return to being the person you used to be. Realize that your old self served you in the best way possible *then*. What you need now is something different, even if you're not exactly sure what that is. Keep venturing with courage and what you seek will become apparent.

Eventually, people will adjust to the emergence of your "self." Some will take it in stride. Some will leave you. Others will come who were not in your life before. These new friends actually like people who say no. They are attracted to people who know who they are and act on that in a way that is both respectful of self and others. In healthy relationships, each person can be strong without being aggressive and caring without being passive.

Being kind to people who welcome your strength, your real self, is easy. It's also authentic. Authenticity cools the fire of resentment. True love of self and others emerges. Road Rage becomes a thing of the past. The whole thing breeds health.

Gods, Beliefs, Illnesses, and Angers

The power of your beliefs, whether or not they include

some construct of a god or transpersonal force, may be impacted by your *thoughts* about those beliefs. What you believe is not at issue here. *What's important is recognizing the impact of your thoughts about your beliefs, whatever they are or are not.* Your thoughts about your beliefs can be either life-giving or life-taking. Your position on all things, including matters of spirit, and the related thoughts you assign to those beliefs can either help and strengthen you during your illness journey or hinder you. Don't overlook that power. Be conscious and harness the power of your beliefs, whatever they are. Finding more power in the self often means visiting the anger holding the power, whether the anger is at a god, your self, your illness, or any number of other things.

Let me be more concrete. Say you believe there is something deep inside that is wise and guiding you. Maybe you call that God or The True Self or simply the goodness of humankind. Since being diagnosed, that belief may have flourished, and you cherish a profound connection with this inner goodness, or God, or part, however you describe it. You see the presence of that power even in your pain. You can't escape its love. You know way down inside that your God, or this innate goodness, is powerfully on your side. In a sense, your thoughts about your beliefs are strengthening you. This is not just emotional and mental strengthening. A 2001 article in *Neuroendocrinology Letters* suggests that spiritual joy may enhance immune efficacy and slow down tumor growth.[16]

Cool, but here's a look at this matter from another angle. If you're a say-yes adult, your thoughts about your beliefs may not be so uplifting. You may be actually turning around the same beliefs that have strengthened others and pointing them against yourself, through your thinking. For example, perhaps you believe in God. But if you find it difficult to express your anger with people, it may be equally difficult to express anger at your God. This suggests that you think God may punish you for that anger, so you can't really be who you are. Once again, the self is getting stuck inside. You may even think that your illness is a punishment from your God. This is a trick bag that's very tough to escape. At a time when one could use all the support available, a nurturing experience of a god has been taken out of the picture. What may be happening is that God has become a reflection of your human experience. In a sense, God has become limited to what you *think* God is.

So, if your God is punitive because you *think* that way, why not think another way—a way that perhaps supports you? Why not think of God as loving every cell of who you are? Why not think that God, or that deep, wise part of you, enjoys your disagreements? Why not think that God proudly receives the strength of your anger and relishes the thought that you can feel so powerfully? Why not think that God has been waiting for you to be completely honest, to bring your whole self to its loving presence, so God can cradle all of you, so you can feel loved more than you knew possible? You can choose that.

This isn't about conversion or being born again or any of that stuff—not in the conventional sense. But think about it. If you have assigned a tremendous amount of power to some belief, or something, or someone, and then turn that power against yourself by what you think, why not use your thoughts to convert that power back into something that helps you? Your thoughts are more powerful than you recognize. Remember the visualization research cited in Chapter 5?

Learning to Say No

Something said by lots of survivors in lots of ways is that recovery is self-care, not selfish. It's about survival. When you cut your hand, the physical self doesn't ponder whether or not it should use its immune cells to repair the wound. The strong instinct to stay well, to take care of the self, happens automatically. Perhaps herein lies a message to the mental, emotional, and spiritual self. In essence, if you don't instinctively take care of the rest of your self, your emotions and mind may become ill and limited, just like the body would without a similar instinct.

This gets slippery. Most great religions hold selflessness in high regard and teach to love others as the self is loved. They teach that true happiness is found in this way of life. I agree, but only with the whole truth of such precepts. Something very subtle lies in these tenets that often seems underplayed and overlooked. These principles of selflessness assume that *one's self* is truly loved and treated well!

It starts with the self. It's not "love your self as you love your neighbor." You love others only as well as you love yourself. If you love yourself well, you love others well. But if you don't love yourself well, you truly can't love others well.

Another way to think of it is that if you consistently give your self away, there is eventually no self left. What do you give then? We all have met people who seem hollow. They laugh but seem disconnected from their joy. They give but don't really seem present when they do— eyes distant, though looking right at you; mind without focus; body almost hapless. In these people, the self has been completely given away. Even Buddha, Christ, and saints of the great religions found ways to nourish the spirit: time alone, time in prayer, time being cared for by others, even time in anger. When you stop paying attention to your "instinct" to take care of yourself in simple decisions like resting or taking time alone though a friend needs help, you lose a part of your self.

Yes, there are of course times when people give although they don't really want to. However, if you consistently ignore the voice of self-care, you will be injured. No one is responsible for you but you. When you solidly acknowledge that fact, you begin *creating* rather than *reacting* in life. What we create is limitless. Giving by choice from the life you have created generates more life, and not just for you. Others can sense this difference in how you give. Even their reactions add life to yours. To create your life, you need skills in saying no.

To answer the question, "How do you say no?" consider first this question: "What happens when your bucket is empty?" When you have emptied yourself to the point of exhaustion, what do you do? Do you give some more? What does that give you: a sense of self, a sense of mastery, a sense of satisfaction, a sense of safety because you aren't sure what else to do when asked to give? The Need Theorists tell us that all our behavior is motivated by some need. In other words, if you always say yes, there is some benefit in that for you. Acknowledge what that benefit is, and accept yourself completely for it. It's not a matter of good or bad. It's simply who you are today.

If you can identify *the need,* you may then be able to find more direct ways to meet it—ways without the potential toll on the self. Selflessness has its own rewards, but if there is no self left, then there is no real gift either. So many give because they have learned no other way of being. The giving then becomes rote, and rote giving is not really a choice. And the gift is, therefore, not really a gift. When we learn to say no, giving becomes a choice, and then it truly is a gift.

So, one of the best ways to learn to say no is to first listen deeply to the self. Listen for what you really need or want, in all situations. Lots of people don't know how to do this. The focus in early life for these people was always outside the self—what others expected, needed, or wanted.

Tuning into the self in this way takes patience and love. Start with little things like, "What time do I really like to go to bed?" or, "Do I like to be the passenger or the driver?"

As you get dialed in with your self and who you really are, make that known when decisions are being made. You don't have to shout it. No need to whisper. Simply speak the truth about who you are. You'll be surprised at people's reactions when you come from this no-nonsense, gentle power. Hold your ground.

If you do choose to concede in some situation, having made your needs known, that concession will feel different to you. The end result may be exactly the same, but when you say yes after making your needs known, this giving then is a choice and feels that way—like creating—and your heart will not shrink. You will sample the impact that choosing has on your spirit and your self. Choosing and using your power in this way expands the self.

Pay close attention to what happens inside as you start saying no or even in just thinking about saying no. This may give you some information about the benefit you get for saying yes. Let what you feel when you start to say no inform you. Notice who, where, and when saying no feels better and when it feels worse. Lastly, don't be surprised if you get a bit carried away with saying no. Think about a pendulum between the two extremes of always saying yes and always saying no. If you have more often than not said yes, when you start saying no, that pendulum may swing all the way to the other side before it finds a natural place somewhere in the middle.

Conclusion

Returning to the story of Francie: She eventually befriended the anger she found inside. Once she had an internal reference for anger, she discovered the anger showing up in her life in lots of little ways...and some big ways, too. As she became skilled at acknowledging her own anger, she worked to accept it. And this was work. The anger scared and confused her. Feeling angry seemed so foreign. She wanted to retract from this unfamiliar feeling. Since her external personality was so fashioned as a woman who didn't get angry, accepting her anger was like rebuilding the self. But she kept accepting.

Eventually, something curious happened. Her voice could be heard, literally and figuratively. Francie would come to session reporting instances when she found herself feeling angry during the previous week. More and more, she responded to those instances by expressing her disapproval. She said people would look at her funny, like, "Who is this?" But she liked respecting herself in this way. In time, relationships started to change. Her parents began treating her differently. The people she worked with also treated her differently. Her inner landscape was different. She was beginning to reshape her life and she liked the shape of it.

The power held in her anger was emerging—not always perfectly, but it was emerging. Over the months, Francie became more and more effective with her power. Her life, as she said directly, felt better. Her life was teaching her that the more one lives in healthy power, the less one lives in anger, hurt, and fear. Conversely, the less one connects with healthy power, the more one lives in anger, hurt, and fear. And making contact with that wonderful, healthy power, lying in wait, often means *going through* the anger, hurt, and fear also waiting. Here's another opportunity to create the rest of your life. What will you make?

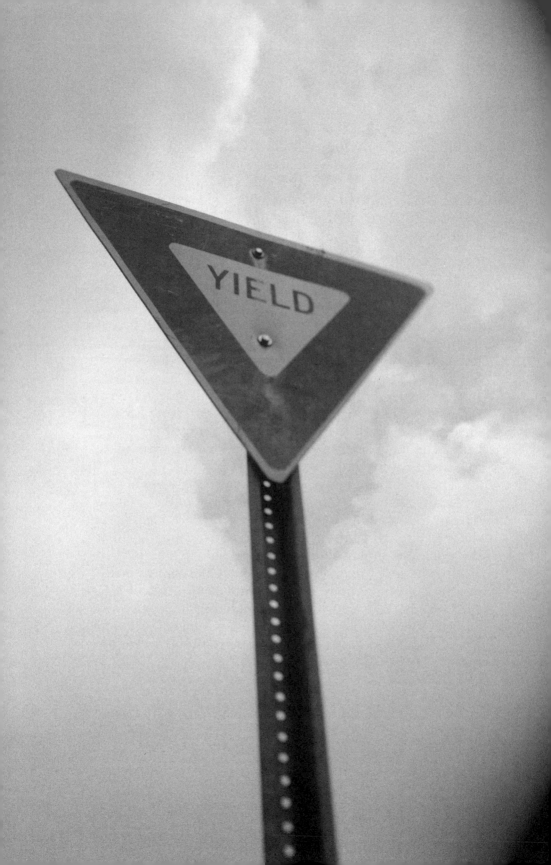

Chapter Twenty-Two

Rest Stop #8: Move with— An Exercise in Resolution

ou've been in the car a long time together. If you are learning and practicing the art of saying no, things may be getting a bit tense in there, especially if the important people in your car—your life—are used to you saying yes. You can actually work this out without pulling off the recovery road and without giving your power away. Here's one approach:

Move With—An Exercise in Resolution

Step 1. Put your ego in your pocket
Step 2. Acknowledge through a sentence what was said to you
Step 3. Ask for more information

Remember the show "Kung Fu?" Couldn't miss it when I was a teen. Remember how the masters would stand nearly motionless while under attack, but opponents would fly? How did the masters do this?

Essentially, a master would move with, rather than against, the opponent. The master would redirect the force brought by the opponent to neutralize the attacker.

For example, if an attacker rushes the master from the front, the master turns slightly while pushing the passing attacker lightly in the same direction the attacker is moving. This well placed and gentle push is enough to create imbalance in the attacker. The master stays relatively still. The attacker is put off-balance and then easily neutralized. The master does not attack back. That non-offensive tenet is central in many martial arts. It's not about winning. It's about neutralizingand then resolving without harm. Aggression is frowned upon and used only in the most extreme circumstances. A quiet mind is the master's weapon...and peace the victory.

You have probably already begun to make the translation from fistfights to verbal ones. When someone takes a verbal swing at you (criticizes you, minimizes you, won't listen, laughs at you, etc.), you may be inclined to play along or go off on that person: say yes or say no aggressively. Neither brings much resolution. There is a middle ground where you stand firmly, but don't get drawn into a shouting match.

During the illness journey, especially if you've been traveling together with someone a long time, it is human to have relationship tension. Nerves get frayed and things get said. Here's an example of how that can go:

Verbal punch: "I can't believe you're still in bed. I know you're in treatment, but come on."

Counterpunch: "Would you just get outta here. You don't have a clue what this is like."

Punch again: "Who needs a clue! Anybody could tell you're spending too much time in bed."

At this point, blood has been drawn. People have been hurt. So how can martial arts be applied to this kind of stressful communication? Sometimes *move with* your opponent.

Step 1. Put Your Ego in Your Pocket

This is the simplest of the three steps but by far the most important and the most difficult, especially if you're learning to say no. When you **put your ego in your pocket**, you decide that loving is more important than winning. This may sound smaultzy, but the consequences of this simple decision can be profound. It doesn't mean, to be sure, that you ought to always put your ego in your pocket. Sometimes making yourself heard, getting angry, or saying no, even though others disagree or seem uncomfortable, is exactly what's needed. But other times, you may choose another style of intcracting. There is always the power of choice.

In thc style of communicating suggested by this Rest Stop, the first step involves checking yourself. And putting your ego in your pocket can be very painful. Your pocket may not be big enough. Besides that, anything but fighting back may feel like giving in, not respecting the self, losing face, or giving power away. So often fear of losing power or some sense of mastery is what ongoing arguments are about. And, of coursc, these escalating arguments are more akin to talking to a drunk—"Forgetaboutit." The real point gets lost in the emotion after tempers flare.

So the first step in breaking this pain-producing cycle is for somebody to slowly back away from the need to win or control the other: ego, pocket. If this is a practice unfamiliar to you, it could feel like your relationship is going to cave in—scary. And don't expcct the other person to get it right away. You've been sparring together this way for a long time: you punch, they punch; they punch, you punch. Be prepared for adjustment time. Putting your ego in your pocket is the relationship equivalent of the martial artist standing in potent stillness and not fighting back. This is power and mastery of another sort.

Step 2. Acknowledge Through a Sentence What Was Said to You

Back to the punch: "I can't believe you're still in bed. I know you're in treatment, but come on." Here's the *move with* part. From your stillness, you are prepared not to attack back but to move with: to practice a different step. When attacked, the master gently redirects the attacker's force so as to neutralize. What's the relationship equivalent? A verbal, martial arts response to the verbal punch described above might sound something like this: "It's hard for you to see me sleeping so much."

Spouse drops mouth open. Why? Not from your punch but precisely because this response isn't a counter-punch. This response focuses on the attacker's message, not a comeback, and *moves with it.* The "It's hard for you . . ." statement acknowledges without agreeing. It *is not* saying, "You're right. I spend too much time in bed." It *is* saying, "I'm not interested in winning or fighting back. Nor am I interested in agreeing or conceding. I am interested in making this better and maybe even learning from it. And to start with, I want you to know I heard all of what you said." That's a lot.

The verbal, martial arts response **acknowledges through a sentence what was said** by the "attacker." You, the "attacked," simply do your best to rephrase the thoughts and feelings communicated by the attacker. You gather up the heart of the message sent your way, and with honest interest, you send a message back that says, "I get it." This way, your response moves *with* the attacker, rather than *against*.

Gotta have your ego in your pocket to do this. Nice

thing is, if it works, the other person may start trying to communicate with you in the same way. Long-range result, you both feel heard more often. Sometimes that's enough.

Step 3. Ask for More Information

To make it clear that you're not just using some technique, it helps to follow at this point with a question. So after responding to the verbal punch above with, "It's hard for you to see me sleeping so much," you might add a question like, "What is it about my sleeping that bothers you?"

Now, if you're doing this for real, you might find that the other person responds to your lovely question with something like, "I'm frustrated! You don't do a thing around here." Well. Hmmm. Boy.

OK, so you have a choice now. You can take that ego back out of your pocket and attack as well: "And do know how many times I've said that to you?!" On the other hand, when the person counters with more "attacking," it is possible to go with another round of Steps Two and Three: "Man, you are really steamed. What has you so upset?" Presentation is everything. No sarcastic tones or nasty faces.

I was waiting one afternoon to meet with an organization leader who supervised staff that he asked me to monitor. When he arrived late for the appointment, he pointed to a chair in his office and literally said, "Sit!" He slammed the door to his office so hard that pictures crashed to the floor. He then proceeded to launch a verbal assault on a report I had given him. While strongly tempted to counterpunch, I decided to instead use Steps Two and Three in some form or fashion. Then he stopped dead in his tracks, explained what he had just come from, and apologized for his behavior. It was then that he could actually hear me.

So, when attacked, you always have the punch back, block, duck and run options. Or you can try this new stuff. For example, after grinding through the sleeping dialogue as outlined above, a caregiver might reveal that he or she is *also* completely exhausted. With that information, together you can fashion a way to get the caregiver some rest.

Or how about this solution? It may become clear that your caregiver really doesn't get your fatigue or its power over you. So, together you decide to talk about this with your nurse the next time you go in for treatment. There are many other possible reactions at this point that could actually lead to some troubles being resolved. Yeah boy.

But you really have to be committed to improving the relationship. You have to choose a time to practice this technique when you have the necessary strength. Or you can go about business as usual. It's yours to decide.

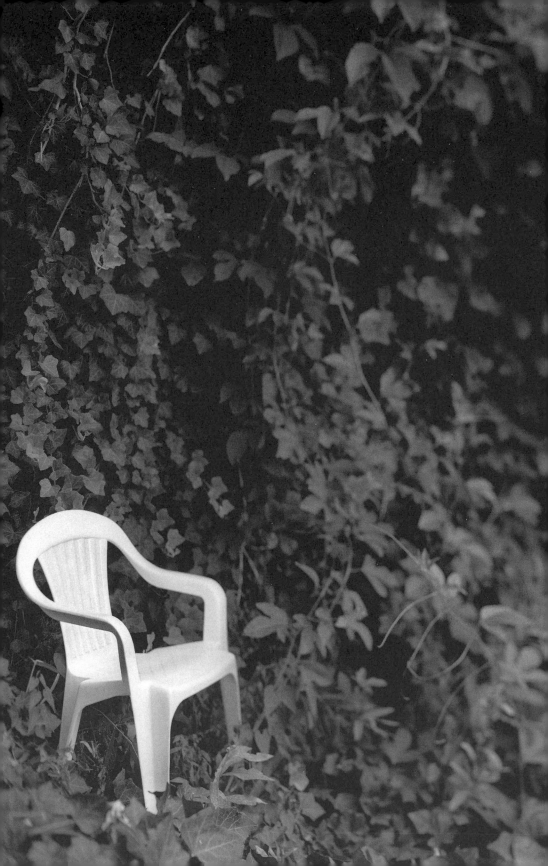

Chapter Twenty-Three

Driving Alone: Changes in Your Support System

You, the survivor, and those who love you have logged many hours on the road. But now you're getting better, at least physically. The crisis is over. The focus that came early on, the newness, the start-up activity of the journey are long past. The routine of treatments and/or follow-up visits may be lulling everyone to sleep. Everything is OK, right?

Well, sooner or later, the people who have been supporting you and your family may begin to nod off one by one. They may feel they were there for the tough times. They were. And you are very glad they were. But now, the greeting cards have stop coming. The phone calls aren't as often. One part of you is glad. Some other part may feel something other than glad.

And before saying any more about losing support, it's important to acknowledge—as a survivor attending a presentation recently pointed out to me—that not everyone dealing with illness has travel companionship to lose. If you are one of those survivors who has been on the journey beyond diagnosis alone, your road has perhaps been especially trying. Hopefully, this book provides you some support. The resources at the end of the book may provide a bridge for you to ongoing contact with others dealing with the same thing you are. Telephone calls and e-mails, if nothing else, may be highways to less isolation.

Returning to those survivors who may be losing support, you might start to feel alone with your illness, and you're not sure you're ready for that. If you are the care-giver or the medical professional, you may feel you have to pull this weight alone: nobody around to hear of your continued discomfort.

For the survivor, a spouse or best friend is usually the last to go. Just like driving, they want to stay awake with you, but eventually even they may slip into sleep. They really don't mean to. But those lines on the highway keep coming: "You're counts look good," "Come back to see me in three months," "I don't need to see you for a year." That is fantastic news. Yes, it is. But you may not be fully recovered emotionally.

Unfortunately, some of your supporters may just feel that they can't give anymore. They, too, are emotionally spent. They need rest. They may feel they have gotten as close as they can. They may have their own emotions and family issues. And so you're alone at the wheel.

Solitude has its own power. If you can find that power, driving with everyone else asleep is much more doable. There are some very useful tools out there designed to help find power in solitude. Many of these tools can guide you through an inner journey, using your mind and active imagination. These approaches are similar to those mentioned in Chapter 5. You'll find some of these tools listed in this book's bibliography.

Like rest stops along the highway, these tools may leave you refreshed with a clearer mind. If you've had support all along, the solitude may be exactly what you need right now. It's OK. After the quiet time—the time taken to be with your own spirit, thoughts, and feelings – the road will still be there. This isn't a race. It's a journey.

Chapter Twenty-Four

Rest Stop #9: Sleep and the Racing Mind

hy is it that falling asleep behind the wheel is something you may have to fight, but falling asleep on your own pillow sometimes seems impossible? It has to do with brain wave activity, and this chapter will explore a simple exercise to capitalize on this brain function notion to help you fall asleep more quickly.

Anxiety, as we've discussed throughout this book, is one of the most common emotions experienced during the journey beyond diagnosis. Anxiety would generally be considered a fear-based response. Although fear, like so many difficult emotions, is often thought of as negative, it, like all emotions, is intended to inform us. Without fear, all of us would constantly be injured, physically and emotionally.

Fear is like a car alarm. It tells us when something is not right. Thank goodness for this warning system. However, significant anxiety is like a hypersensitive car alarm: it goes off unnecessarily, eventually becoming a nuisance rather than an aid.

For a lot of survivors and caregivers who are trying to fall asleep, the racing, anxious mind is like the car alarm that just keeps going off, making it impossible to rest. What's this about, and why is it so much easier to get drowsy behind the wheel?

First of all, the racing mind, like the oversensitive car alarm, is just doing its job. It's simply doing it too well. Mental activity is often an attempt to create firm ground on which to stand. During an illness diagnosis so much

happens and changes. Nothing seems stable. By constantly turning thoughts, situations, and experiences over and
over in the mind, the mind is trying to order an otherwise
chaotic-feeling circumstance. This organizing function
comforts us and helps us live more productively. But
when the mind won't stop organizing, grinding, and racing, something very uncomfortable and unproductive
occurs, especially when trying to sleep. The racing mind
becomes too much of a good thing. With a habitually
racing mind, the organizing thought process has become
a kind of addiction—an attempt to make you feel better
that actually harms you in the long run.

So, it's not a matter of stopping the mind from activity but stepping it down gradually to a lesser rate of activity, like managing withdrawal for the addict.
This step down process is what happens on the highway.
The mind trains itself—busies itself if you will—on
the passing posts and white lines. The mind then
gradually lets go of racing as it shifts into watching the
environment. This simple mental focus that happens
automatically on the highway is the basis for most
meditation techniques. The mind continues to be active,
but at a much simpler level, and brain wave activity
changes and slows.

Did you know that Einstein's theory of relativity came
to him in his sleep? How many times have you woken up
with a solution to a problem? Have you also noticed that
many "solutions" seem to just show up
in your mind, when you're doing something besides
thinking about "the problem?" This is good reason to let
your mind relax, especially when trying to sleep.

It appears that a racing mind simply cycles the same
information over and over. With so much activity, there's

rarely room for any new information to surface. And yet, when we sleep or focus on other things, the information around "the problem" settles and even reconfigures itself, leading to new ideas and the emergence of something completely different. This is the creative process, and an effective approach to problem solving.

The point here is that a running, non-stop mind produces very little to help fix the actual problem or perceived concern that the mind is churning to resolve. So, instead, why not try the following exercise when attempting to fall asleep. It gives the mind something else to focus on, like passing highway lines do. And who knows, with the mind quiet, some real and useable information might surface that may actually help with the "problem."

At this point, I'd like to suggest that you read the rest of the chapter. When you're finished, you can either record the script suggested in the following section and replay it when it's time to sleep or have someone else read the script to you as you fall asleep.

Sleep and the Racing Mind

Step 1. Breathe and be gentle with your mind
Step 2. Return to your body
Step 3. Plant yourself

Step 1. Breathe and Be Gentle with Your Mind

As we said earlier, a racing mind is indicative of anxiety, and anxiety is a fear-based response to life. Fear-based responses are designed to protect you. As such, fear-based responses actually gear you up. To do that, fear-based responses release chemicals in the body that ready it to fight or run. So could this be any more contrary to what you want when you lie down to sleep? Have you ever noticed when trying to fall asleep that, after a while of the racing mind, you just feel like getting up and doing something? That's exactly what the chemicals released in the body during a fear-based response are designed to do: initiate action.

The body's call to action is generally accompanied by rapid and shallow breathing. The shallow breath supports the body's release of action-oriented chemicals. And the more chemicals released, the more shallow the breath, and the more shallow the breath, the more chemicals released, and so on. That's when you jump out of bed. Sleep, you know at this point, is impossible.

So, there are three key ingredients in this buildup to action, when all you want to do is fall asleep. There's the *mind racing* to create a sense of order during a time in your life that feels chaotic. There's the *shallow breathing*. Finally, there's the *release of action-oriented chemicals* in the body. Believe it or not, you have the capacity to address all three of these ingredients. By consciously shifting the racing mind and the breath, you can alter the body's release of action-oriented chemicals. So let's start by shifting the breath.

The first part of Step 1 is simply to BREATHE. When you become conscious of your breath and begin to slow it down by breathing deep, full breaths, you are sending a message to your body that says, "It's OK. At this moment, things are alright."

If you do nothing else but take deep, full breaths, you will begin to change your body chemistry. Your body will begin to feel, "It's OK to just lie here. Fighting or running is not required right now." That may sound strange, but if your breath has been shallow, your body thinks it's preparing for action. Changing your breath can change the quality of your thoughts, and your chemistry.

The second part of Step 1 begins to more directly address the thinking process. Steps 2 and 3 will continue a change in your thinking process, but Step 1 begins that shift in a very important way: BE GENTLE WITH YOUR MIND.

What does it mean to be gentle with your mind, and why is it important? If your mind tends to race, that "habit" *isn't* going to stop over night—no pun intended. You've been operating in the world in that way for years. So, be patient as you try some other way. And remember, when your mind races, it's trying to help you. Your mind wants to create the feeling of mastery over the troubling situation.

So as you move into Steps 2 and 3, your mind may have a tendency to get off course and start to race again. That's OK. Gently invite your mind to return to the thoughts suggested in the next step. If it helps, speak with your mind: "I know you want to help me by racing to solution, mulling over the situation again and again. But when you race, my body gets charged up, and I find it difficult to settle down. I want to settle down. I trust that any improvements I might make in my situation will become clear to me, even if I stop thinking about them right now. So thank you for trying to help, but what I want and need right now is to return my mind to the thoughts suggested by this exercise."

Why is it important to be gentle with your mind? If you start getting frustrated with the fact that in the middle of this exercise your mind wants to race again, you might set up a win-lose situation inside your own head. It can happen when you turn this exercise into a task *you must* successfully complete. When that happens, you may begin to speak to your mind with demands like, "You will stop racing. I will go to sleep." Most of us tend to resist demands, even when they come from some part of ourselves. At this point, it's as if one part is saying, "You will sleep," and another part responds with, "I don't think so," or, "You can't make me." Then you're stuck. You can avoid this win-lose by not demanding that your mind perform but by inviting it to slow down. Not only that, if you demand that your mind slow down, and your mind has trouble satisfying this demand (because going slow has not been your mind's norm), then you might get *anxious*, which fuels the release of those fear-based, action-oriented chemicals. Now you're up again.

Step 2. Return to Your Body

Everyone knows that the human body carries an electrical charge. It's this charge that fires across nerve endings and gives rhythm to the heart muscle. That's why medical professionals use paddles that send electricity to the heart when it stops.

Science tells us that whenever an object carries an electrical charge, there is an electromagnetic field in and around that object. Because the human body does carry an electrical charge, there is then an electromagnetic field in and around it. This "field," which may be stronger in some, has been depicted in art for thousands of years, often as a halo or radiance around the body of mystics, masters, and saints. Many cultures over the centuries have developed ways to work with this field for the purpose of health. Today, the National Institute of Health is studying contemporary techniques developed by medical professionals who balance and strengthen this electromagnetic field in and around humans to support wellness, happiness, and wholeness.

The human electromagnetic field is egg-shaped, with the larger end around the shoulders and head, and the smaller end at the feet. Consider that when your mind is racing, there's a lot of electricity firing in and around your head. Consider that as the mind races, and more and more electricity is generated in your head, your electromagnetic field expands there, evacuating the rest of your body in response to the demands for electricity by the mind. Consider, then, that when your mind races part of you in the form of your electromagnetic field leaves your body to gather up and around your head. Have you ever felt hollow and cold when your mind is racing? Have your legs felt weak?

Step 2 suggests that you **Return To Your Body**. That is, imagine that your electromagnetic field is gently pouring back into the rest of your body from in and around your head. Here's a visualization to help. If you like, after you've slowed your breathing as suggested in Step 1, read the following paragraph to yourself, or have someone read it to you, or record it and play it back when you're ready to sleep. Remember to be kind with your mind if it wants to race as you read or listen:

My mind is racing to support me, but at this point I'd like to settle down and fall asleep. To help me fall asleep, I am taking deep, full breaths. And as my mind and my breath slow down, I am occupying my mind with this image: I see my electromagnetic field like a large soap bubble attached to the top of my head. With each slow inhale, I see the bubble shrinking, as if my inhale is drawing air into my body from inside the bubble.

And as this air from inside the bubble is drawn down through my head and neck, it is converted into a beautiful gold light, like honey. And as I continue to breathe, this honey-like light begins to make its way into every cell of my body, bringing calm and quiet.

First, the honey-like light slowly fills my head, my neck, and my shoulders. As it fills these areas, I feel them relax. Next, the honey drains into my upper arms, then my lower arms and now my hands. And as the light reaches these areas, they relax as if being filled at the very cell with pure love.

Now the honey-like light makes its way into the cells of my upper back and chest, and as it does, I actually feel the muscles there relaxing, receiving the love of this light.

As I breath, the bubble above my head gets smaller, and the honey-like light now drains into my middle back and my belly. It feels comforting. As this honey-light pours through me, there is a release of tension as each area is filled and relaxed.

With each deep breath, the golden light makes its way farther down my body, now pouring comfortably into my lower back, my hips, and my groin region. I am finding myself more and more quiet inside as I watch the golden light move through me.

Now the light is in my upper legs and then my knees, and the golden light is filling the cells in my legs with calm and love, and I enjoy the relaxation. And the honey-light continues to pour down into my shins and calf muscles. And now I see that the bubble above my head is nearly completely gone, *as each inhale has emptied it, and the activity contained there has been converted into a golden light, like honey, now reaching my ankles and, finally, filling me completely. The sensation I'm left with is one of fullness, relaxation, and pure love.*

Step 3. Plant Yourself

Native Americans believe that all things have a principal essence or spirit. The earth, for example, has an essence more like the beat of the heart, slow and rhythmic, like the movement of the turtle, paced, predictable, and deliberate, like the color of the soil, dark and rich, and like the sound of the horse walking.

The essence of the sky is more like the firing of nerve endings, like lightning, quick and erratic, like the flight of the hummingbird, excited, charged and changing, like the color of clouds, light and airy, and like the sound of the wind.

As persons, we also each have a principal essence. Some people tend to be more earth-like; others, more sky-like. One is no better than the other. Both bring unique gifts. Earth people are solid folks. You know exactly where they stand. They are more like the buffalo. Sky people are a joy to be around. They accomplish much. They are more like the fox or the bird.

Nature demonstrates daily the value of balance in all things. Balance between earth and sky brings life. We see this in the cycles of the seasons: rain to nourish, sun to flourish, wind to prune, and cold to transition into new life. Disasters caused by too much sky or rain make the consequences of imbalance painfully apparent. On the other hand, drought is an example of not enough sky.

Balance between earth essence and sky essence in

people also brings life. For example, a person with healthy balance between the essence of earth and sky can be solid in beliefs, but open; can be very productive, and still know peace.

And yet, people with too much earth essence may wish they would be more motivated and sometimes feel stuck. On the other hand, people with too much sky essence often wish they could just relax.

I used to be very much a sky person. My movements were fast, my speech was fast, my stomach was fast, and my mind was always active. My mind and my body used to move a lot when trying to sleep. With time and support, I have found a balance that serves me better. As a result, my movements have slowed, my speech is deeper and more deliberate, my stomach rests, and my mind can be still. Sleep comes much easier.

Given these notions, if you regularly have trouble falling or staying asleep, you may have too much sky essence and not enough earth essence. To increase your earth essence, consider now adding the following visualization to those already suggested above, and **Plant Yourself:**

My body feels full and weighty. The honey-like light has filled me in from top to bottom. The fullness I feel is comforting. I feel loved.

The honey-like light I feel in every cell of my body is now beginning to gather in my feet. Because of this, I feel a subtle pressure in my arches, as this light of love pushes against them from the inside out.

Finally, the weight of the honey-like light pooling in my legs and feet is so present that the bottoms of my feet open, allowing the light to gently ooze out.

I continue to feel great peace, fullness, and love in every cell of my body, as the honey-like light pours gently from the bottoms of my feet, making its way past my bed, through my home to the earth below. As this honey-like light reaches the earth, it begins to turn a darker color, like molasses or deep, rose-pedal red. And as it reaches the earth and turns this darker color, it begins to stretch into the earth, like roots.

These dark roots coming from the bottoms of my feet are reaching deep into the soil. As these roots stretch into the earth, I feel an even greater sense of calm, as if any tension or unwanted activity of mind or body is being pulled down, through my body, and out the bottoms of my feet.

These dark roots continue to stretch farther and farther into the heart of the earth, and as they do, I feel a profound sense of trust, like a tree firmly planted and completely stable. I feel this from the top of my head to the very bottoms of my feet.

And like a tree firmly planted, as the dark roots reach farther into the rich soil of the earth, these same roots begin to nourish me, bringing back to me an even richer sense of love, health, and calm. As these nourishing feelings return to me from the earth, my body responds with pure stillness, relaxation, peace, and comfort. I am finding it easy to begin to slip into a state of rich restfulness.

Sleep is now upon me. I am full from head to toe and in every cell of my body with a sense of profound calm, experiencing deep love in all of me. And the earth is sending even more quiet and compassion into me through the bottoms of my feet. Sleep is here. I am one with all that is at rest.

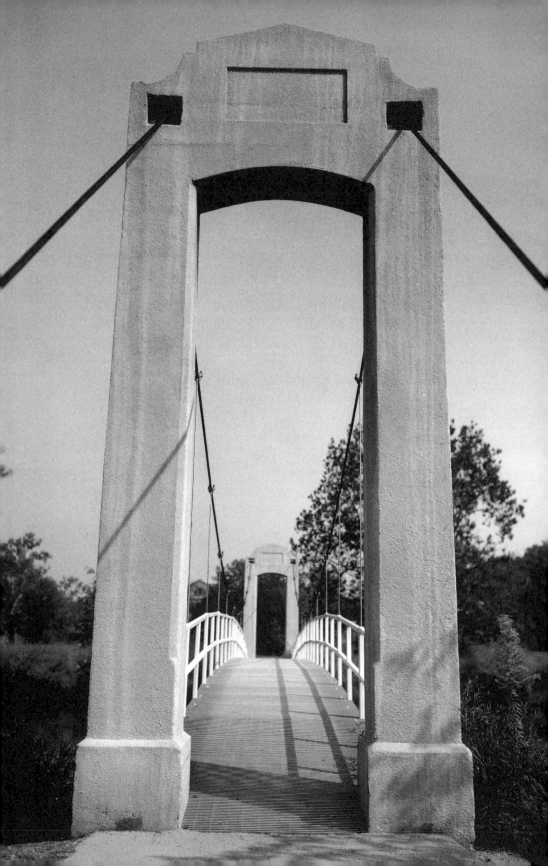

Chapter Twenty-Five

Maintenance: Links of Body and Mind

Throughout this book, and especially in Chapter 5, science and the expertise of highly regarded professionals has been cited supporting the notion that what happens in your heart, mind, relationships, and spirit affects what happens in your body. Science is confirming that throughout the journey of life, when one aspect of the self is maintained, the rest of the self is positively affected. But there are stories with no real scientific support that corroborate the body/mind link: stories of tumors disappearing just before surgery, or stories of countless tumors leaving patients during comas.

To be sure, there are many unanswered questions about physical illness. So many illnesses have genetic and environmental links. There is also the issue of spontaneous remission and miracles. But is there something you can do to promote these wonderful occurrences?

We know through science that, when stressed, we change our body chemistry. If the stress persists, we weaken immune function. We also know that most of the time our experience of stress is a product of what we do internally, with external circumstances. For example, hailstorms happen in the Midwest. If ten people work in an office, and one hailstorm nails all ten of their cars, there may be ten different internal reactions to that external circumstance. Those reactions will dictate the level of stress in each of those ten people.

It's natural to have a reaction when your vehicle gets

pelted with hail. It's honest. But for many, it doesn't stop there. The mind then takes over where the emotions left off. Some folks might relive the hailstorm many times in their heads, perhaps seeking some way to resolve the uncomfortable feelings. Yet, emotions can't be resolved— they just are. So the mind starts to spin, pursuing some mastery of what was once an *external* circumstance that has now become an *internal* situation. The lack of resolution introduces anxiety. This can lead to a racing mind and more tension or stress—the mind is anything but quiet.

On the other hand, when the initial, natural feelings are allowed to just show up and pass through, they dissipate. When you do this, you're basically saying to yourself, "Yes, this makes me mad, and it's going to be a hassle to fix, but I'm alright, even with these feelings and this situation." This introduces trust. The mind is then more quiet.

Trust is good medicine. Quiet minds are trusting minds. This isn't necessarily about trusting anyone or anything. It's just that when you trust, a feeling of "It's OK" can start to replace the "Oh, no" feeling that difficult occurrences may stir. When this happens, hail damaged vehicles create less of a rise in you. Not because you're afraid to react or don't think you should react, but because you honestly don't have much reaction in you. Trust becomes a way of life. It develops over time and becomes self-perpetuating because it feels so much more pleasant. It's not about thinking everything *will be* OK, it's about a deepening sense or feeling that everything *is* OK. The feeling is just in you and almost palpable in the body. Trust isn't a thought; it's an experience.

I was completely surprised one Sunday afternoon

when I came home to water pouring out the sides of my house. First, there was a "Damn," and such. But seconds later, standing inside, water running over my shoes, I was even more surprised when the simple thought came, "I'll turn off the water main and call maintenance." That was it. I called, got out the shop vac, and started to clean up.

By living this way—embracing all, yet staying honest and real—the trusting mind gets very still. The quieter your mind is, the more comfortable you are. That alone is enough. But science is demonstrating an interesting link here: the more comfortable your inner life, the healthier your outer body.

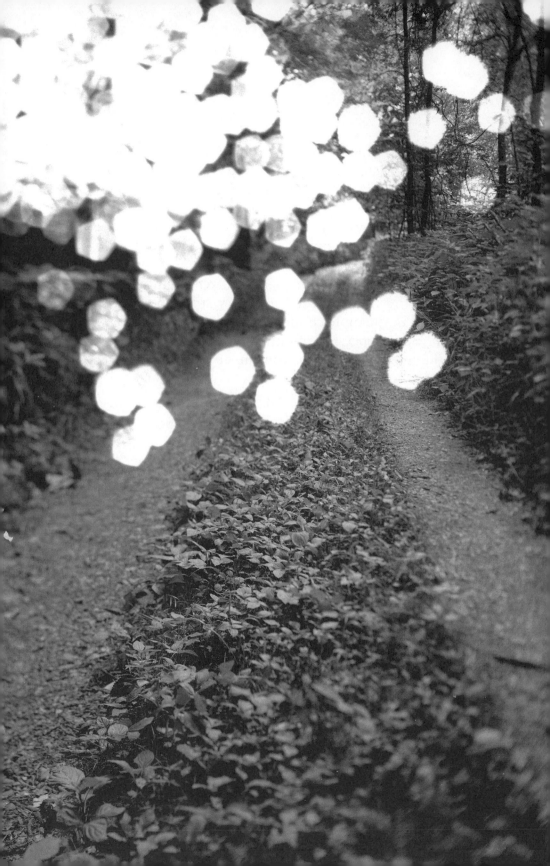

Chapter Twenty-Six

Rest Stop #10: The Road Map of Dreams

Everybody has gotten lost on a drive, some time or another. It's no different with the journey beyond diagnosis, and your own dreams may be the best map back to who you really are. I did my master's thesis on dreams and have worked with dreams for more than twenty years. Dream work is an integral part of my counseling practice. Dreams may tell you more about yourself than any other experience. And even though you may be dreaming about others, it's all about you.

The experience of dreaming cannot be explained or contained in any one theory or even cultural stance. Though the approach that has proven most useful to me is the Gestalt model, I value and sometimes introduce other avenues for understanding dreams.

For example, God, insight, spirit, angels, and all sorts of other holy things have been reported by many cultures over the centuries to show up in dreams. Look at the Torah or the Old and New Testaments. There are tons of stories within about dreams, God, and spiritual influences. And these texts represent only two of the great religions. As we said earlier, Einstein supposedly received his theory of relativity in a dream, and many of you have, no doubt, awoken with solutions. No single theory neatly contains all this, and for me, all possibilities for understanding dreams enhance the therapeutic process.

There is the belief in the Gestalt approach that we all have an instinct for wholeness, and that such instinct shows up most clearly in dreams. Many consider such an instinct sacred. This may sound odd since so many dreams seem anything but whole or sacred.

When you look at the gestalt of a dream, which translated means "whole" or total image, this idea of sacred makes more sense. Take for example the dream of being chased by a bad person. In the Gestalt approach, both the chaser and the person being chased are parts of the dreamer, one part in some way opposed to the other. Consequently, the dream reflects the tension of these opposites. The dreamer's "whole person" is seen in the dream: not just the parts that seem normal and not just the parts that seem scary, aggressive, or abnormal. In theory, such a dream suggests that the dreamer is, at some level, experiencing tension and distance between two opposing parts of the self. The goal of Gestalt therapy is to minimize these kinds of polarities in the self. When that happens, some integration has begun—steps to greater degrees of wholeness. When experienced, this can feel sacred.

When someone brings a dream to therapy, his or her interpretation is always the most important place to start. My work, if agreed to by the client, is to expand what the dreamer finds in the dream. If someone brings a dream and says the dream is an answer to a prayer, then I believe it to be that. If someone brings a dream and says, "I believe this dream is about my relationship with my father," then I believe it to be so. If someone brings a dream and says, "My sister who died four months ago visited me in my dream last night," then I believe it to be that. Sometimes that dreamwork ends there. Other times if the dreamer believes it worth doing, together we may look behind or under or around this initial take on the dream and see if more information may be stored there.

A way into this expanded discussion of the dream is usually indicated by how the dreamer tells the dream. If a character or image from the dream is spoken about repeatedly, that particular character or image probably holds key information. Same goes if the dreamer changes facial or body expressions or tone of voice when talking about a particular part of a dream.

Say you come to a counseling session with a dream. Most people start by describing the dream. Customarily, I will ask you to tell the dream as if you are having it right now: "I am," rather than, "I was." In this way, the dream becomes more an experience and less a report.

What follows is your presentation of the dream: "This is a strange dream. I'm walking through the attic of this old house. I think it's the house I grew up in. I really liked that house, but I didn't like the attic, so it's weird that I'm in that part of the house." You then pause. You look up, slightly pained. Five or six seconds later you get a little smile and say, "I had such fun times with my brothers and sisters in that house. We used to chase each other all over the yard. . . . Anyway, I'm a little spooked about being in the attic. Not as bad as I was as a kid, but a little skittish. This is where it gets strange. All of a sudden, this trap door opens just in front of me and I just miss falling in it." At this point your eyes widen: "Scared the dickens outta me. I think I woke up right after that. I was kind of shaking."

If you offered no interpretation of the dream, I might begin a Gestalt exercise like this: "You have the house, and you have the attic, and you have the trapdoor, and you have you. These seem to be key pieces from the dream. Did I miss anything that's really important to you? OK, then of these pieces, which is *most* important?"

Say your name is Kim, and you brought this dream to counseling. In response to my question, you say the trap-door is the most important piece of the dream. With that, we begin: "I'm gonna ask you to play-act a little with me. This is your dream and your experience. I'll follow you. All right? So in the Gestalt approach, every part of the dream is representing some part of the dreamer. If that's true, one way to find out what each part means about you as the dreamer is to give each part a voice. The play-acting we're about to try is designed to do just that. Ready to give it a try? OK, as odd as this might seem, I want to speak with you, as the trapdoor. What I'd like you to do is move to someplace else in the room where you think the trapdoor might show up. Once you're in that new place, I'm going to have a conversation with you as the trapdoor."

Let me interrupt the dream interaction briefly. First of all, in the dialogue that follows, I am going to press Kim a little more than I might typically, for the sake of education. Secondly, something curious and powerful happens when you ask a client to take up a new position in the room for such an exercise. I've had clients, by choice, act out flying dreams by lying somewhere in the office. Others have crouched away from me, faces hidden, beside a bookcase or chair. Still others have sat in a corner wrapped in the quilt available on my couch, becoming children seen in dreams.

What seems to occur with this relocation is that the aspect of the self represented by a dream symbol separates more cleanly from the rest of the self. When given its own voice in this new position, separate from the rest of the self, the dreamer seems more comfortable letting the symbol speak with its own voice, its own thoughts, and its own feelings. The dreamer's conscious mind is then left more with the dreamer, and not with this now available individual aspect. Consequently, when this aspect that has separated from the dreamer speaks, the words come more freely—less filtered—and therefore more authentic and believable. The dreamer seems more willing to just let this part talk, and new information breaks out.

Back to the dialogue: Kim has decided to stand in the center of the office, like a trapdoor in my floor. So I say to Kim, "Now in this place, you are the trapdoor. I want you to talk in first person as the trapdoor, like you, as a trapdoor, can speak. Like you, Trapdoor, have a voice. Trapdoor, what should I call you?"

Kim says I should call her, as the trapdoor, "No Good."

So we begin our dialogue: "No Good, as a place to begin, would you describe yourself?"

"I'm about this big, and on the floor of the attic, but I'm filled with darkness," Kim says, as the trapdoor.

I say, "No Good, would you say that again?"

Kim repeats, "I'm about this big, and on the floor of the attic, but I'm filled with darkness."

I then say, "Would you repeat just that last part, No Good?"

"But I'm filled with darkness," Kim says.

Then I say, "No Good, would you share more with me about your darkness?"

"The darkness . . . ," Kim starts.

I interject, "My darkness . . ."

"OK, *my* darkness is very thick," Kim explains. "I scare people because of it, just like I scared Kim in the dream. People are afraid to get close to me because of my darkness."

"No Good, say that last sentence again," I request.

Kim explains, "People are afraid to get close to me because of my darkness." At this point, Kim tears up—something has begun to move.

So, that would be our initiation into this dream. With care, I would likely invite Kim to explore the surfacing emotion. Later, in that same session, I might have Kim speak to No Good, the trapdoor, or I might have Kim become the darkness. The process unfolds itself in this way, led by the cues the client leaves. As you see, this approach is not about "interpretation"; it's about letting the dream and all its players speak for themselves. Through this process of dialogue, the parts get to know one another, and the dreamer comes to know the self. In the dream example cited above, what theoratically could unfold are the parts of Kim that are unknown and scary—the trapdoor and its darkness—might make contact with the parts that are more known, life giving, and perhaps filled with light—the parts that provided the courage for Kim to venture into this emotional place. This begins the journey to integration and wholeness.

You might say, "Well, Kim was just making all that stuff up as the trapdoor." You would be exactly correct. And if we gave the same setup to five different people and asked each of them to become the trapdoor, we would have five very different responses, beginning with the name they might choose for the trapdoor.

As a result, the dream characters and all they share are *about the dreamer* and nobody else. The pieces come together very quickly and often with much emotion. Doors open to understanding. With understanding comes a stronger sense of choice. And while sometimes opening us to a degree of internal strife, the outcome often means a fuller sense of self, and more life.

Having said all that, here's a Nine-Step approach for using these concepts to work with your own dreams:

Step 1. Identify the part of your dream most important to you—probably the part that comes to mind quickly or the part you feel strongest about, either positively or negatively.

Step 2. Identify the significant "character" from this important part of your dream. This character can be a person, an object, an animal, or even a feeling or sound.

Step 3. Give this character a name. If the character has a real name like Nancy or Spot, you can use that name or you can use a name that more closely fits what you felt in the dream about that character. Let this name come from your gut, not your mind, e.g., Ugly Creature or Angel Voice. Use any name that speaks to you—Wise One, Broken Down Car, White Horse, or Precious Child, etc.

Step 4. Fold a piece of paper in half and write your name at the top of one column and your character's name at the top of the other column.

Step 5. Write a script between you and your dream character, listing responses under the appropriate name on your divided page. A good place to start is for you to say to your character, "Describe yourself to me." For example, if your character's name is Broken Down Car, it might respond to your opening question with something like, "I'm big, but I'm kind of a wreck. There are holes in me." And you might respond with, "What happened to you?"

Let the dialogue continue freely and without filtering until it feels finished. BE SURE THAT EACH OF YOU SPEAKS ONLY IN FIRST PERSON, i.e., "*I'm* kind of a wreck," not, "*It's* kind of a wreck."

Step 6. This step is necessary only if something uncomfortable happened in your dream that you're still uneasy about. Find some time to be quiet and go back into the dream. See it as if it was happening right now, but use your power to recreate the uncomfortable dream experience in a way that supports you or makes you feel better, i.e., you outrun or overpower your attacker; you sprout wings and fly before you hit the ground. Try not to get stuck within these "recreations." Do what comes naturally, and if you struggle to resolve the situation, breathe compassion into yourself, and try again later. These are only images intending to teach you.

Step 7. Now, put your dialogue aside for a few days; a week or more is OK. This distance created by time helps shake any literal translation you might still hold to. Then *read only the words under your dream character's name.* As you read these words, they should be in first person, like, "I'm a white, powerful horse. I am strong and full of life," or, "I am only two years old, and because I have no legs, I can't stand on my own." Read those words again, out loud.

Step 8. Write down any of your reactions once you've read your character's words out loud.

Step 9. Consider these questions: Does this dream have anything to say to you? Do the words from your character remind you of any part of you? Does the feeling you have when reading your character's words resemble the feeling of any part of your life today? How might this information impact how you choose to be in the future?

You may find these nine steps useful in tapping a truly powerful resource. The wisdom, guidance, and truth offered by your dream life can be potent and healing. This built-in therapy is available free every night. You get to let this map guide you to your True Self and to greater wholeness.

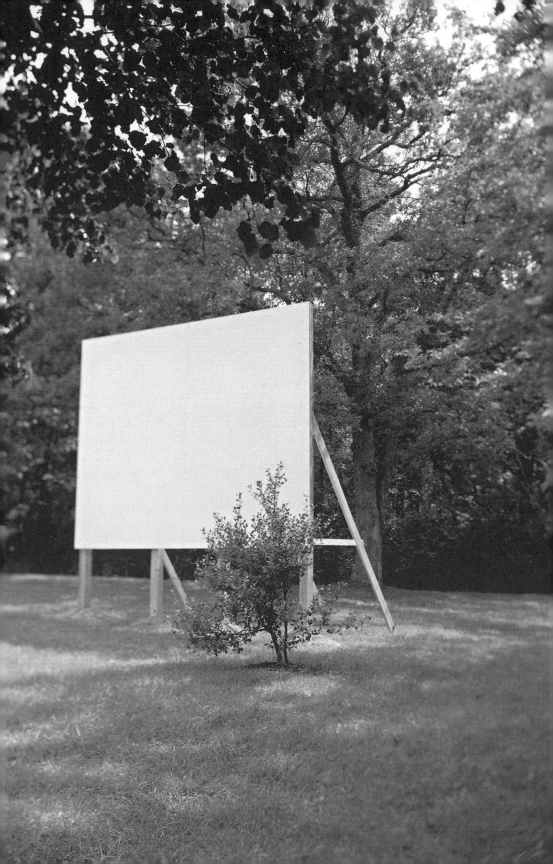

Chapter Twenty-Seven

Nearing Your Destination: Signs You're Getting Close

*I*s greater integration the goal of your journey beyond diagnosis? What about a quiet mind? How about health and joy? Or do you seek improved relationships? Perhaps you're after parts of all these intentions. What is your journey's destination? It's different for everyone, and with any long trip, you'll see signs when you're getting close.

As you approach your destination, you may notice more happiness in your heart or more trust in your relationships. You might discover that your attention is returning to the rest of life—the parts that were background earlier in the illness journey are now more foreground. You may find that the first thing you think about in the morning is not your illness. You may notice that ads for illness-related drugs, or "walks," don't stir you up like they use to. You might realize a freshness in your spirit. Your actions may show that you value something today that is different from what you valued this time last year.

Excellent, but a note of caution. By saying there is a "destination," you instantly create good, better, and best destinations, like vacation comparisons. Then, of course, there will have to be good, better, and best ways to *reach* that destination. When that happens, you set up the possibility of judging or being judged for the progress, style, or quality of your journey and your destination.

What if there was no best destination—just the one

you hoped for and wanted? What if you traveled toward that destination with trust? What if in traveling with trust, your hopes and wants gently changed and developed along the way? What if you found that way of traveling gratifying?

Here's a curious twist. Have you ever just taken off in your car, not knowing where you're going. What a fascinating way to head out on a Saturday morning. This kind of "travel" can be extra relaxing. In those glorious hours, something lovely happens. It's now just about being. And in just being, every goal for that drive is satisfied. What an interesting way that would be to live. It's the difference between living in trust and living in fear. The destination may be very similar, but the spirit with which you travel can make the journey itself quite different.

Speaking of spirit, this chapter wouldn't feel complete without letting you in on a secret of sorts. It's been my privilege to lead hundreds of support group meetings for hundreds of men and women surviving illness and their caregivers. My ears have heard many precious stories, thoughts, and feelings in these most honorable exchanges. My eyes have witnessed courage in the face of pain or evey kind: body, mind, and spirit. People in these groups have wrestled with the greatest of demons. All have come face to face with death, and some felt its breath. Many knew they were dying, and did. Over months and years, individuals and entire groups have painstakingly peeled through layers of humanness.

Many peeled back the layer of power. Others prestige. Some dug through the layer of wealth and possessions. Beneath those, some ventured past layers of "friendship," and even family and faith. Finally, health, hope, pain and life itself were scrutinized, analyzed, and peeled away. Ane the one thing that remained, the one destination more often sought by travelers on the journey beyond diagnosis, was love. Love–to love and be loved.

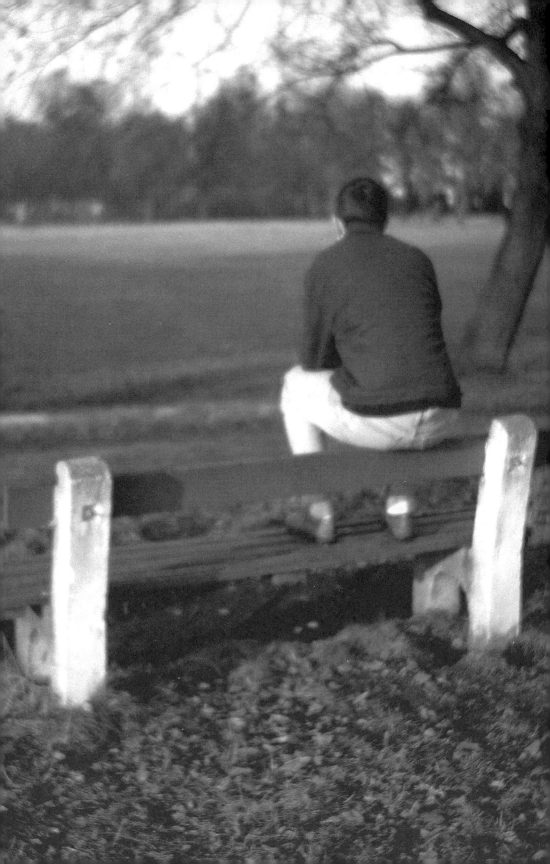

Chapter Twenty-Eight

The Journey Continues: Ongoing Survivorship

For many, physical well-being is the destination of the journey beyond diagnosis. When health is recovered, life returns to normal, and maybe it even improves. With better health, these sojourners go forward with renewed gratitude, reconfigured values, clarity, happiness, and hope. And for many others, the journey ventures past the goal of physical well-being. These travelers, too, have been deeply affected by illness. However, once physical wellness is recovered, they continue to travel, in a mindful way. This leg of the trip is now sharply focused on recovery of relationships, the mind, and the spirit.

This ongoing travel may be difficult for some to understand. When treatment ends, or when the five-year survivorship mark is reached, everyone celebrates, including the survivor. And yet for many survivors these events are not the end of the journey.

A middle-aged gentleman got his support group's attention one night with these thoughts: "In just a few weeks, it's gonna be five years since they told me I had lung cancer. I'm doing really well, and I'm thankful every day. But I still need to come to this meeting once a month."

"'Still need,'" I said. "That suggests that you shouldn't need."

"Well," he shared, "it helps me to be around people who know what it's like, but my wife doesn't seem to appreciate that."

"What tells you she doesn't appreciate that?" I asked.

"When I was getting ready to come tonight," he said, "she asked me where I was going, and when I told her, she just kind of walked away from me. I asked her what was wrong and she said, 'I don't know. I guess I don't understand why you still need that group.'" In sharing this, his slight hesitation suggested some emotions were showing up.

"What effect do those kinds of comments from your wife have on you?" I asked.

Though it was tough for him to speak, his words found their way out: "Sometimes I feel alone in my own home."

To be sure, many people are very happy to forget the entire illness experience. For others, there is a continuing concern that the illness experience will never be forgotten. Then there are those who never want to forget because of all that the illness experience helped them learn. They intentionally remember it, so as to maintain new ways of life that serve them better. Many who believed they would never be free of "illness thoughts" find they can go a long time without them. I have actually met survivors and caregivers who completely forgot about the illness.

But, then there are times it can be difficult to think of anything but the illness: diagnosis anniversaries and check-ups. These moments in the continuing journey can be especially difficult. There may be a wave of emotion when returning to the doctor's office, even years after treatment has successfully ended. Too, lots of scary thoughts and memories of the "early days" can pop up for survivors and caregivers during the time surrounding anniversaries. You might call these *occasion reactions*. If someone is having one of these *occasion reactions*, it only makes things worse when others say things like, "It's just another routine check-up," or, "Why are you still getting upset about this?"

These *occasion reactions* provide a perfect opportunity for practicing self-care and effective communication. If you are the one having the *occasion reaction*, but not feeling supported, acknowledge what you feel. You have a right to ask for what you need. Teach the one you want more support from to ask you who, what, where, when, and how questions at anniversary or check-up times: "How are you doing with the upcoming check-up?" or, "What effect is this diagnosis anniversary having on you?" In teaching others these skills, you are being responsible for yourselves.

If you're supporting someone having an *occasion reaction*, listen with your heart and question with love. Simply be present, not to resolve but to learn. Ask questions in an authentic, open way, without accusation. Ask those open-ended questions, and then practice the simple but powerful art of golden silence. Try not to turn your questioning into an interrogation or a lesson on how to get over the illness. If you see patterns in the answers, share them with the person you're supporting, when it helps.

If you haven't been diagnosed with an illness, you probably really don't understand. If you haven't been the primary support person to someone diagnosed with an illness, you probably really don't understand. As hard as it may be to comprehend, the survivor or caregiver you love may need support about the illness for years to come. It can be an opportunity for both of you to gain a deeper knowledge of one another, thereby deepening the intimacy you share. The journey continues. See what you can do to improve the ride.

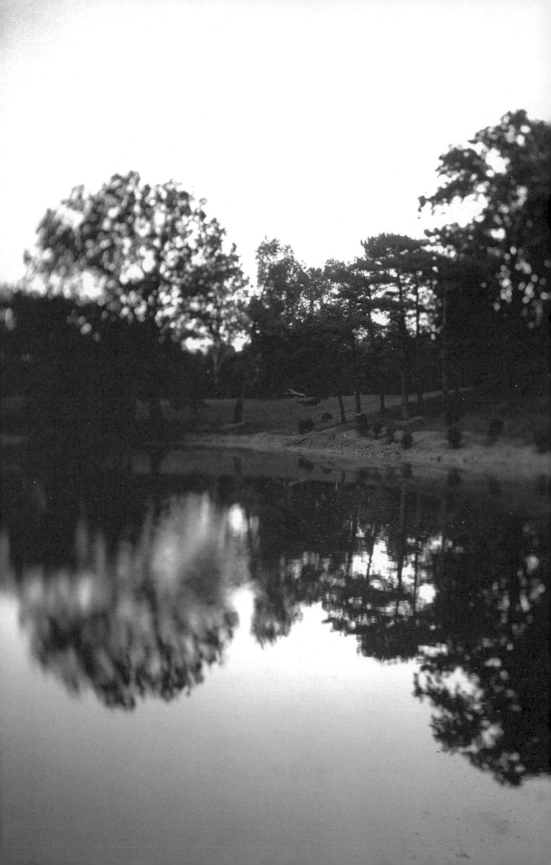

Chapter Twenty-Nine

Beyond the Mountaintops: The Journey of Death and Dying

While tremendously courageous in their travels, there are, of course, those who do not survive their illness, and the current human journey comes to an end. While these loved ones may find exceptional degrees of emotional, mental, relational, and spiritual health while they are dying, their bodies steadily decline.

To those survivors whose bodies are in decline, respect this part of the journey as you have all others and ask those supporting you to do the same. You may decide to stay in some form of treatment, even unto death. So be it. This is an honorable choice. Or there may come a time when you choose to discontinue treatment. Let it be so. This is an honorable choice. Know that whatever you decide is exactly the right thing for you.

If you can, make decisions about how you want to die (e.g., when or if to use life support, etc.) while your mind is still clear and capable. If you worry that you won't be able to tell when your mind is failing, let your family or someone you strongly trust know that you are worried. Then ask them to tell you when they see the very early signs of your mind weakening. This way, you will know it's time to address big decisions, if you haven't already.

Whatever you decide, some will support your choices and some will not. If you decide to continue treatment until death, some will say, "You shouldn't put yourself through that," or, "Why are you still holding on to some shred of hope? Why can't you just let go?" Remember, it is your journey, not theirs.

If you decide to discontinue treatment, some will say, "You shouldn't give up. There's still hope," or, "My illness is worse than yours. I would give anything to be in your shoes. And you want to stop treatment? That's not fair." Remember, it's your journey, not theirs.

Choosing to stop treatment is just that: a choice. It's not necessarily giving up. It may be a very solid, well-thought-out, and determined decision. It may simply be, in your mind, the best choice, all things considered. This choice may scare some of the people around you. It may force them to look more closely at the reality of the situation. For some illness survivors, your choice may also get them thinking about an option they are not quite ready to consider: a choice that makes them very uncomfortable. Their uncomfortableness may look like anger. But choice is still yours.

By the way, *giving up* is also a choice. But giving up has such negative connotations. Maybe we should call it giving in. Or surrendering. Or simply *giving*. That may say it best for some people—giving peace to one's own heart and the hearts and spirits of those who love you.

Twilight

Twilight is that time between stages of light at day's end that changes the way things look. During the twilight of life, things start to look and feel different. Twilight during the journey beyond diagnosis happens when dying becomes more imminent. Twilight occurs in a few ways. This time between life and death can begin subtly, when the survivor starts to contend with multiple recurrences or complications. Of course, recurrences and complications don't automatically mean the survivor is on a sure path to death from the illness. And yet, during these times, the survivor and those supporting the survivor may have fleeting thoughts about the possibility of death. This can be an unusual period of continued hope and quiet grieving.

The other occasion of twilight is when the survivor is more definitely approaching death. This is the time when all recognize that the survivor is probably going to die from the illness. The transition from more hope to less hope ensues. The shift from less grief to more grief unfolds.

Curious behaviors may surface in family and friends. Some involved with the illness survivor may begin to race about trying to stop the sun from setting. That is, trying to halt what is inevitable—the death of the one they love. This can be unsettling as these people hold fiercely to any thread of hope. That's how the love is often expressed in those last moments of light: bringing home news bulletins about potential "cures" and last-ditch-effort approaches—and bellies full of pain. But the sun continues to set.

In time, though, often following the lead of the survivor, one by one, those who love the survivor surrender to their own longings for hope and ease their wrestling with the sun. Acceptance is dawning. At this point, waves of hurt overtake. One person is affected, and then feels better for a time. Then another person feels the waves crash. Families can get confused by this rhythm of pain. A member of the family may be in a place of deep hurt in the morning, but much better later that same day. Or someone else will be all right, but that person's spouse is struggling in the waves of hurt. It might begin to feel like roulette, never knowing who's going to be OK and who's going to want support.

Some supporters attempt to change themselves with each changing set of circumstances and emotions. Be only who you are. Your journey has been long, and the toughest roads are just ahead. When you find something pleasant, enjoy it. At a time like this, the spirit absolutely needs refreshment. Somehow there's a belief that you must be in as much pain as the dying person. Be assured that if you are an honest human being, you will have genuine pain. That is enough.

Follow the dying person's lead. If he or she wants to talk, then listen without the "It's gonna be OKs" and "Don't talk like thats." If the dying person wants to go on with life as best he or she can, try to go along. At the same time, don't completely cut yourself off from the pain of your own truth.

The natural, emotional trauma of watching someone you love die can be unbearable. Some respond by pushing even harder against the sun, demanding that the survivor try this, or go there. Sadly, the person dying now is burdened with this caregiver's needs. Sadder still is the pain of the person who clutches to the one dying until the very death.

Death and Fear

Say goodbye to each other with as much grace as you can and while you still have the chance. Don't miss the opportunity to stand before your dying loved one with all that you feel. This may also invite the one you love so much to do the same. In this place of authenticity you can both connect heart to heart. If you battle against the sun to the very end, you leave little room for an honest good-bye. Your spirit is unavailable to the spirit of your loved one because it is occupied by fear. A final goodbye is powerfully painful. Fear makes it worse. Wouldn't you much rather release each other's hearts from this life with love?

There was a young woman in a group who had a great fear of death. She was devoted to her group for years. During that time she witnessed the dying of several group mates. Eventually, the young woman began missing group meetings because of her own illness, but she would always call to explain her absence. One week she didn't show for group, but there was no call. So someone in the group decided to call her and report back at the next session. At that next meeting the group found out the young woman had been raced to the hospital and nearly died.

But the young woman did eventually return to her group. Everybody wanted to know what happened. It seemed some rare complication struck hard, and she was not expected to survive. Because the young woman had spoken at length about her fear of death in previous meetings, the group wanted to know what it was like for her to nearly die. Immediately, her arms went straight up over her head, hands wide open. Then, with a clear, quiet, soulful smile, and looking right into the heart of the group, she said, "Like letting go. Like putting your hands in the air at the top of the roller coaster." In that instant for her, death became something very different.

Death for Tibetans brings with it what they refer to as a *Bardo*. According to this tenet, death creates, for anyone involved, an opportunity of tremendous spiritual movement. If an illness diagnosis opens the window to greater truth, then death opens the door.

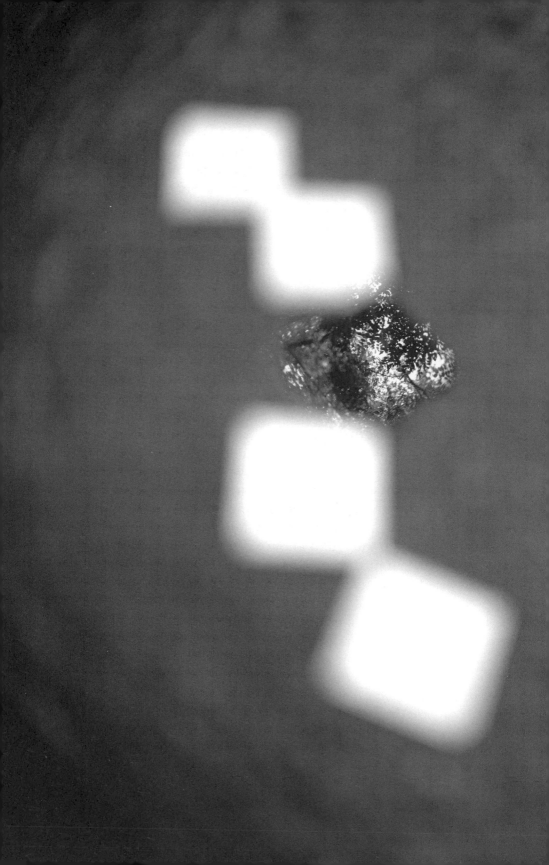

Chapter Thirty

Further Destinations:
Matters of Spirit

egardless of the physical outcomes from an illness journey, matters of spirit can surface for all involved. An article from *Issues in Mental Health Nursing* tells us that spiritual well-being may be an important internal resource for persons forced to adjust to un certainty related to long-term health problems.[17] Given that kind of data, I speak directly in this chapter of spirituality, especially surrounding questions of pain, death, and the loss of physical life.

In the last chapter, we introduced a Tibetan notion called the Bardo: the opening to matters of spirit for anyone exposed to a death experience. Death has been a regular part of my work with the chronically and terminally ill. Many illness survivors have allowed me into the final days of their journey. Many caregivers have let me stand beside them as they make their way beyond the death of the one they loved. These times have always brought deep stirring in some mysterious place in me.

This is a place we all have. It would be impossible for any person profoundly connected to another person by pain and honesty and hope and courage and real joy not to be in some way moved by that person's death. This isn't about feeling the dying person's pain, or getting lost in the loss. When repeatedly a part of this life/death dynamic, professionals working with disease survivors are often greatly affected at the level of beliefs and values. Curiously enough, great hope may be gleaned from these encounters.

Three of the most well-known contemporary experts in the mysteries of death and dying have all found hope laced through their work. Raymond Moody, Jr., MD, PhD, Brian L. Weiss, MD, and the late Elisabeth Kubler-Ross, MD, all do or have believed without hesitation that when the body dies the spirit lives on. Moreover, the state of existence the spirit comes to after it leaves the body is filled with truth and love and light. These hope-filled conclusions are the product of thousands of interviews these experts have conducted with individuals who have had near-death experiences, or near-death-like experiences, during regressive hypnotherapy.

In one of his groundbreaking books, *Through Time Into Healing*, Dr. Weiss writes, "It is important to keep an open mind, to trust your experiences. Don't let the dogma and beliefs of others undermine your personal experience and perceptions of reality." [18]

Much has been written about death and dying, and the written word can teach. But experience changes everything. With enough experiences about life and death that go beyond what can be known with the mind, beliefs shape themselves. And life changes. Life expands.

I will always remember the first time I actually saw light around a dying person: a young man in his early thirties. He had been away from his weekly support group for a while because he was so sick. He came back to say goodbye. A beautiful, soft light was apparent around him. He died in love the next week. Days later, I was struck by the same light around a baby. It dawned on me that the baby had just come from the light, and the young man was being drawn back into it. The great poet William Wordsworth tells us, "Heaven lies about us in our infancy!" That exclamation point is his.

Many caregivers have returned to their groups reporting that their dying loved ones were heard to be talking with deceased friends and family members, reaching for them, or asking others in the room if they had seen these visitors. This is very consistent with the findings of Dr. Moody and others. Many surviving near-death experiences report being greeted upon their own death by loved ones that have died before them.

Other mystical experiences are not uncommon for the dying. A lovely woman was nearing death but still attending her weekly support group. One day in group, she began to stare up, moving her head as if tracking something high above her.

"What do you see?" I softly asked. The group was a bit taken by her behavior.

With an ever-so-slight smile she quietly answered, "Eagles."

"Eagles carry the medicine of Great Spirit, according to Native American tradition," I offered. Her smile widened, and later she shared how comforted she was by the Native American belief. She died the next week.

With the gift of traveling beside hundreds of survivors and caregivers, over miles and miles of roads on the illness journey, it is difficult not to see all as holy. Even death. We do our best to push against death and pain of all kinds. Yet, pain is firmly rooted in the human condition. It is hard to communicate how much *life* pours from rooms filled with illness survivors and caregivers, many in real pain or dying. These people come to these rooms with all their pain and their hope and their fear and their courage. And there, in that way, truths appear. In facing death, many see life for the first time.

Even death can give life. I remember a middle-aged man who was dearly loved by his group. Having missed many meetings without word from him or his family, the group believed he had died. We then spend the better part of a session saying goodbye. Each member, in turn, expressed what the man had meant to him or her. Much rich emotion and honesty rose up from the group. It was real. It was powerfully alive.

The next week, oxygen in tow, the man returned to the group. The group was awestruck. He, too, had come back to say goodbye. The group proceeded to say to him directly what had been said in his absence the week before. With the dying man's permission, each group member spoke to him from someplace way inside. Then the man spoke, eye to eye, with each group member. This was a divine moment. After addressing each of his fellow members individually, he spoke to the group as a whole: "I've waited all my life to know I meant something to someone. Now I know I do."

Near the close of this most poignant meeting, the man apologized to the group for exposing them over the last few months to the details of his dying, which included all sorts of practical questions and ethereal concerns. The group did a direct and effective job of releasing the man from his concern. Then the words of a very young member made their way straight to the heart of this matter: "Your journey has shown me sign posts along the way of death, so when that time comes for me, I will be more ready. Your grace in dying has given me hope."

After the meeting, I was debriefing with a young co-leader—someone who had been personally struggling with questions of religion and spirituality. With eyes wet immediately, the young therapist said softly, "God was in there." I couldn't agree more.

Not only did dying not diminish the presence of love in these weekly support groups, it was in the very tension, torment, and truth of the dying process that I witnessed many *gaining* on life. This gain occurred not just with the dying members, but also with the surviving group members who saw more clearly what held value in the human experience through the dying and deaths of those they had grown so intimately connected.

Love never dimmed. That's not to say that group members were willing to face the death of their group mates with arms open. Of course it was hard. That love, too, was real and holy. Love cannot be bettered by pain or death.

Shaped by these experiences, witnessing the death process time and time again, something changes inside. Seeing so much light coming from and through the journey of dying, the darkness our culture ties to death gets released. Life and death become different parts of the same wave. When deeply rooted in the security of this knowing, those of us still in body are empowered to branch further into all that human *life* offers. We know humanity, pain, confusion—we know darkness—to value the light. Cultures that embrace death and dying, rather than push against it, live with balance. Farmers understand this.

Having been so shaped by experience, I am filled with broadened beliefs. It is my belief that the most important part of each of us lives on beyond the physical form. This brilliant essence (call it the soul) is evolving through life in each of us. In our purest form, we are compassion. We come to human life by choice and as an act of compassion. There is a most holy Source Of All compassion, and each of us is a glimmering facet of that Source—one with It, yet separate. As such, *each of us created* the blueprint for this life before we came, *not God or our parents or anyone else*. We, like moths, seek more light. The world is a place to find out about light, truth, love: what expands love and what contracts it. With this developing awareness, our light grows. Soul growth is instinct of the highest form. Through life, we grow into as much of who we really are as possible. And even more of who we really are will become visible later.

Could it be that each person involved with the illness journey chose that road, as a compassion-filled soul, before birth, through an act of love and desire for deeper understanding? Did the one diagnosed with the illness take on the most physically challenging part? Has each person in the journey evolved as a spiritual being? Through this united gesture of souls, have all those connected to the journey beyond diagnosis offered powerful and healing knowledge to all others?

Illness opens the individual (both human and soul) to things before unseen, unfelt, and unknown. Collectively, this is power for transformation. Might it be so that all the people, with all the horrible illnesses, have been changing the world through their pain? Is this dynamic at work in all life journeys, whether painful or joyful? And what if death was simply a transition, not an opponent to be beaten? Where would we put all the joy and the hope and the peace? In the human experience, journey is the destination. Journeying is life. The human experience is part of the soul's journey. What if all this is part of the greater journey of man?

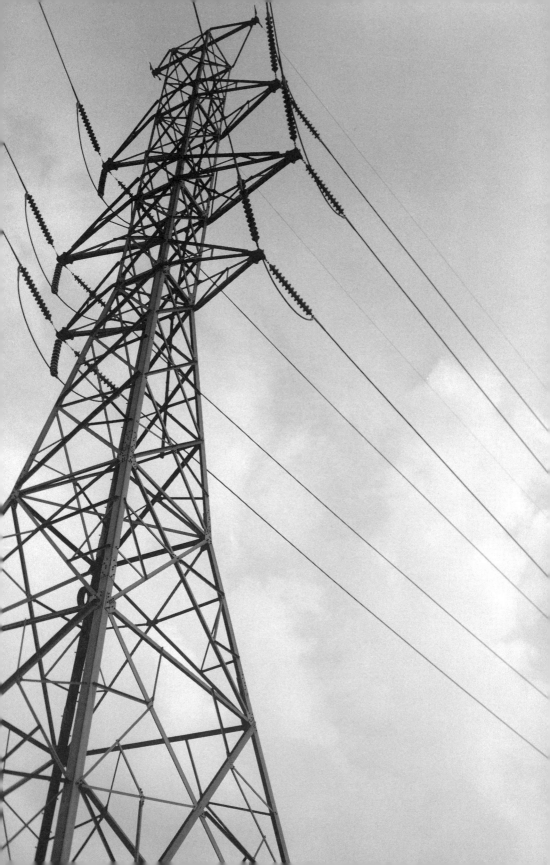

Chapter Thirty-One

Rest Stop #11:
Staying in Touch

*W*hen someone you love dies, it is natural to want to stay in touch with that person. In ancient times and cultures, this desire to maintain contact was seen as normal. Spiritual traditions were developed to actually support that contact. What's most curious is that modern science may be proving the validity and power of these ancient ways. A principle bridge between ancient traditions and modern beliefs was Einstein's work. His theory of relativity led us to understand that, at its simplest level, all is energy. Einstein's work opened the door to quantum physics and other contemporary physics which suggest that if all is energy, then all is connected—an energetic web of sorts.

One striking example of the "all is energy" notion is the quartz watch. The watch is powered by a *rock* that emanates some useable form of charge or energy. Instruments are now being tested that measure a similar charge or energy emitting from nearly everything, including the human being. It stands to reason that if a rock emits energy, so might a living organism. Actually, EKGs and EEGs measure the electrical impulses of the body that carry messages across nerve endings and fire the cadence of the heart.

If, as Einstein postulated, *everything* is energy, you can deduce that *all aspects* of the human—our bodies, our thoughts, our feelings, (our souls?)—produce energy as well. It is common knowledge and solidly documented that everybody, regardless of age, weight, size, race, religion, gender, or sexual persuasion, loses the weight of five nickels at the instant of death. That weight loss is identical for all. Many believe this to be the weight of the soul—the weight of that part of us that is, was, and always will be.

If it's true that all bodies, thoughts, feelings, and souls are connected by a kind of energetic web, then "movement" on any one part of that web would be detected by all other parts. This is one explanation for intuition and ESP. It also explains the power of the ancient, mystical ways used for staying in touch with loved ones, *whether the loved one was living or dead.*

To explain how this "energy web" might appear in the everyday, here's a simple case study from just this week. A client had recently been exploring the impact of fear in his life. In this particular session, we began to discuss the flip side of fear. I posed: "If fear was on one side of a coin—like the head on one side of a coin or penny was fear—and things like confusion and doubt made up the background around that head, what would be on the other side of that coin, and what would make up that background? Isn't it wheat on the back of a penny?"

Now that's a mighty convoluted question, but it seemed like the words weren't even out of my mouth when the client exclaimed, "I can't believe you just talked about what's on the other side of a penny! I had a dream last night about finding coins, and I was trying to figure out in my dream what was on the back of a penny!"

Since I had never, in more than twenty-five years of counseling, used the penny for any kind of analogy, and certainly never questioned a client about what was on the back of a penny, I immediately thought about the energy web. Had he moved the web in his dreams the night before with curiosity about the backside of a penny, and then that "movement" registered with me in our session the following morning? Furthermore, was it coincidence that I decided to add this chapter to this book the very week that this penny incident occurred?

This isn't magic. This isn't voodoo. Perhaps coincidence. Or perhaps it's just the truth according to modern physics. Fortunately, lots of cultures didn't and still don't need modern physics to support their ancient and continued practices that reflect these now- researched phenomena. And fortunately for cultures like ours, modern physics is opening us back up to these possibilities.

There's a fascinating book called, *Kything: The Art of Spiritual Presence*, by Louis M. Savary, STD, PhD, and Patricia H. Berne, PhD.[19] The book explores some of the ancient ways for staying in touch with people separate from you by space or time and offers many techniques. Einstein and today's physicists completely support this space-time construct.

Many who have lost a loved one often long to share special occasions with that person. Others wish they still had that loved one to help with tough decisions. There are those who believe without a doubt that their dead loved one is still with them in spirit, and even guides them. Many fall asleep telling their loved one about their day. This is natural and, given the solid ground of modern physics, perhaps more real than we first believed. There is, of course, an equally natural grieving process that fosters an often painful but healthy separation from the loved one. Grieving is the subject of many other books. The following exercise is designed to bridge that mourning process and support the nearly automatic communication that often continues between loved ones after a death.

The exercise is a hybrid approach combining ancient ways, communication skills, and human electromagnetic field techniques like those now being rigorously studied at the National Institute of Health and widely practiced in hospitals across the United States and around the world.

Effectiveness of the following technique may be bolstered when those interested in using it come to an agreement about its potential before attempting to practice it. Also, anyone who has or is being treated for a dissociative disorder should consult a professional before attempting to use the following exercise:

Staying in Touch

Step 1. Open your heart
Step 2. Invite your loved one
Step 3. Listen
Step 4. Release in love

Step 1. Open Your Heart

Any time we seek effective communication, openness helps. It's no different when hoping to communicate with someone without the use of electronics or the five senses. In addition to being open to what the other person says, feels, or believes, this exercise includes being open at the heart and self, energetically. Try not to let this language spook you. Instead, let the experience support and teach you. We're talking here about creating "movement" on the energy web that we described earlier. Again,

Einstein's work and contemporary physics show us that *all* is energy.

To open the heart and self, find quiet. In the quiet, imagine being able to see the energy that is you and everything else. See that energy in your mind's eye as it quickens every cell of your body. You may see it as billions of particles of light or feel it as a deep and subtle hum in and around every part of you. Simply allow whatever image or experience comes to you representing this all-pervasive energy.

Now, imagine that with your simple wish this same energy in and around you and everything else can gather and flow through you as a healing force. With this imagination, what do you see in your mind's eye? Is this healing force flowing in through your head or your feet? Perhaps you feel a vibration. Trust whatever image or experience comes to you. Ancient and modern religious traditions from Christianity to Judaism and Hinduism to Buddhism have found varied names for these kinds of happenings. None of this is new to man.

Now, ask for that healing force flowing into you to gather in your chest or belly, whichever feels more comfortable to you. Allow this place to be filled with this tremendous healing power. Take a few deep breaths as you imagine this pooling.

Step 2. Invite Your Loved One

Whether the loved one you wish to communicate with is living or dead, invite him or her to join you. Start by inviting that person to open his or her self in the same way you just did. Keep breathing. Now send a flow of the healing power pooled in your chest or belly to your loved one and invite him or her to send a flow to you in the same way.

If you both agree, allow those flows to connect. Breathe.

Step 3. Listen

Now that you have established a connection with your loved one, simply listen. Like any communication, listening is usually the best place to start. Allow any dialogue to develop naturally. Be yourself.

Step 4. Release in Love

When you agree with your loved one that it is time to conclude your communication, in a very gentle way each of you draw back the force of healing to the self. When you feel that you and your loved one have both recovered your own healing force, let that healing force comfort you as you release each other in love, regardless of what or how you communicated, knowing you may reconnect whenever you agree to that.

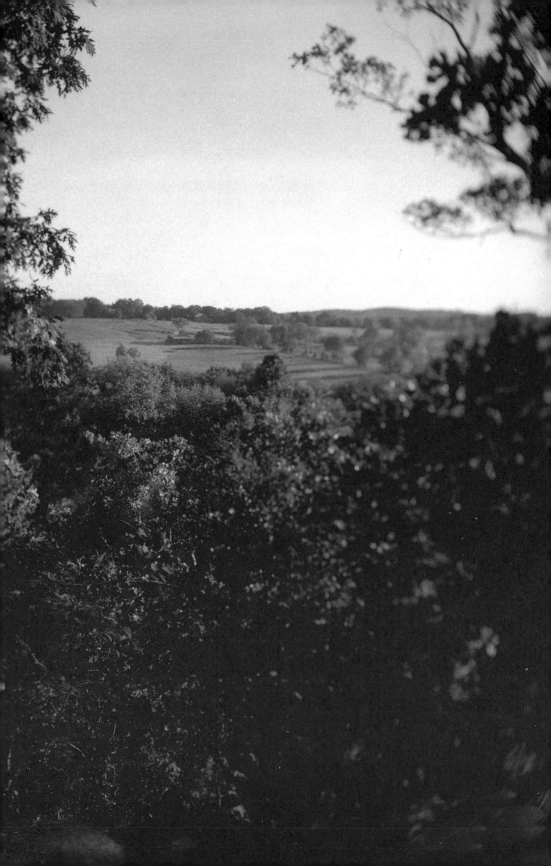

Chapter Thirty-Two

Bon Voyage

So the time has come for us to continue on our own unique and separate journeys beyond diagnosis. In wanting to wish you a meaningful farewell, my words have seemed lacking. And then there was a message from Joey.

Joe is a twenty-six-year-old man with severe autism. Along with many other physical complications resulting from this diagnosis, Joey has extreme apraxia: a neurological impairment that essentially has the affect of crisscrossing and disconnecting nerves, making signals from the brain to the body jumbled and confused. For those with this malady, the simple act of pointing takes concentration and effort—even facial muscles find it difficult to respond naturally and fluidly to thoughts and feelings. The body cannot do what the mind asks. Consequently, Joey's first steps came at the age of nine.

Another result of apraxia for Joey is that he only now, and with great celebration, speaks two or three words. When very young, Joey was diagnosed as severely mentally retarded. However, this young man, his mother, and his family would not accept that diagnosis. For many years, varied treatments and approaches were laboriously explored.

Imagine being perceived by most as retarded, taking in information for twenty-four years, possessing a brilliant mind but having no way to express that brilliance.

And then in 2004, through the persistence of this young man and the people who love him, Joe was introduced to facilitated communication—a technique used by occupational therapists that supports the hand of nonverbal, autistic children and adults as they point to letters on a large alphabet board.

Through facilitated communication, with focused attention on his own hand, Joey began directing his supported fingers to letters. Very quickly Joey had "a voice," and what he spoke was astounding. Some believe that many autistic children and adults are shrouded mystics. Joey, for me, fits that description.

Several people have been trained to use facilitated communication with Joey. And while the facilitators change, the spirit, message, syntax, and articulations from Joey remain constant. Over the year since he found his voice, Joey has changed. In the beginning, he expressed pain and anger, for good reason. Then the flavor of his expressions began to shift. Now, he delights like never before. His external emotion is matching the emotion he communicates through his spelling. It appears that communicating all he has held inside is adding to Joey's life. Some who learn facilitated communication eventually manipulate a conventional keyboard unassisted.

As for Joey, he hopes to "mouth talk" one day, and that day is upon us. And as for me, any form of communication from this young man goes right to my heart.

And so it became clear, in receiving his most recent message, that Joey's words—the words of a "fellow traveler"—could speak to you in ways my words could not. It is now my distinct honor to share passages from the writings of this gifted soul and bid you bon voyage:

My moment of waltzing in the world of autism is being challenged as I yearn to come out of silence to waltz with words. I lived in a storm of loneliness. Now I am not alone.

I am too morose for words.

I pretend I am not autistic.
I feel trapped in my body.
I touch tomorrow's dreams

I understand more than people know
I say nothing because I can't
I dream I can say something
I try to talk to Mom
I hope my family knows I love them

I am happy now.

Host of stories lurking in my mind
Stories about curse of rigid body and blessings of
flowing mind.

Friends, hug your hearts each time you want to cry

Listen outside of head to know how to heal autism.
Joe makes peace outside of head—in heart.

Friends' abundance of love awaits us in excess.
Friends' abundance of time reveals instantaneousness of love's
embrace.

Fellow travelers behold my name is Joe
My message is hope
Fellow travelers behold

Hope insists its urgency upon our souls
Hope insists its urgency upon our broken bodies

Roadside Assistance: Resources for You and Those You Love

ALS Association, National Office
27001 Agoura Road, Ste. 150
Calabasas Hills, CA 91301-5104
(818) 880-9007
www.alsa.org

Alzheimer's Association
225 N. Michigan Avenue, Ste. 1700
Chicago, IL 60601-7633
(800) 272-3900
www.alz.org

American Amputee Foundation, Inc.
P.O. Box 250218, Hillcrest Station
Little Rock, AR 72225
(501) 666-2523
www.americanamputee.org

American Brain Tumor Association
2720 River Road, Suite 146
Des Plaines, IL 60018
(800) 886-2282
www.abta.org

American Cancer Society
1599 Clifton Rd., N.E.
Atlanta, GA 30329
(800) ACS 2345
www.cancer.org

American Chronic Pain Association
P.O. Box 850
Rocklin, CA 95677-0850
(800) 533-3231
www.theacpa.org

American Diabetes Association
1701 N. Beauregard St.
Alexandria, VA 22311
(800) DIABETES
www.diabetes.org

American Dietetic Association
120 S. Riverside Plaza, Ste. 2000
Chicago, Ill 60606
(800) 366-1655
www.eatright.org

American Fibromyalgia Syndrome Association
6380 E. Tanque Verde Rd., Ste. D.
Tucson, AZ 85715
(520) 733-1570
www.afsafund.org

American Foundation for Urologic Disease
1000 Corporate Blvd.
Linthicum, MD 21090
(800) 828-7866
www.afud.org

American Heart Association
7272 Greenville Avenue
Dallas, TX 75231-4596
(800) 242-8721
www.americanheart.org

American Liver Foundation
75 Maiden Lane, Suite 603
New York, NY 10038-4810
(800) 223-0179
www.liverfoundation.org

American Lung Association
61 Broadway, 6th floor
New York, NY 10006
(800) LUNG-USA
www.lungusa.org

American Parkinson's Disease Association
1250 Hylan Blvd., Ste. 4B
Staten Island, NY 10305-1946
(800) 223-2732
www.apdaparkinson.org

American Society of Clinical Oncology
1900 Duke Street, Ste. 200
Alexandria, VA 22314
(703) 299-0150
www.asco.org

Arthritis Foundation
P.O. Box 932915
Atlanta, GA 31193-2915
(800) 283-7800
www.arthritis.org

Autism Society of America
7910 Woodmont Avenue, Ste. 300
Bethesda, MD 20814-3067
(301) 657-0881
www.autism-society.org/

Candlelighters Childhood Cancer Foundation
P.O. Box 498
Kensington, MD 20895-0498
(800) 366-2223
www.candlelighters.org

Chronic Fatigue Immune Dysfunction Association of America
P.O. Box 220398
Charlotte, NC 28222-0398
(704) 365-2343
www.cfids.org

Chron's and Colitis Foundation of America
386 Park Avenue South, 17th Floor
New York, NY 10016-8840
(800) 932-2423
www.ccfa.org

Corporate Angel Network, Inc.
1 Loop Road, Westchester County Airport
White Plains, NY 10604
(914) 328-1313
www.corpangelnetwork.org

Genetic Alliance, Inc.
4301 Connecticut Ave., NW, Suite 404
Washington, DC 20008-2369
(202) 966-5557
www.geneticalliance.org

Healing Touch International, Inc.
445 Union Blvd., Suite 105
Lakewood, CO 80228
(303) 989-7982
www.healingtouch.net

Hill-Burton Free Care Program
Health Resources and Services Administration
U.S. Department of Health and Human Services
Parklawn Building
5600 Fishers Lane
Rockville, MD 20857
(800) 638-0742
www.hrsa.gov\osp\dfcr

AIDS Info
P.O. Box 6303
Rockville, MD 20849-6303
(800) 448-0440
www.aidsinfo.nih.gov

Hospice Education Institute
3 Unity Square
P.O. Box 98
Machiasport, ME 04655-0098
(800) HOSPICELINK
www.hospiceworld.org

Multiple Sclerosis Association of America
706 Haddonfield Rd.
Cherry Hill, NJ 08002
(800) 532-7667
www.msaa.com

International Myeloma Foundation
12650 Riverside Drive, Suite 206
North Hollywood, CA 91607-3421
USA
(800) 452-CURE
www.myeloma.org

Leukemia and Lymphoma Society
1311 Mamaroneck Avenue
White Plains, NY 10605
(800) 955-4572
www.lls.org

Lupus Foundation of America, Inc.
2000 L. Street, N.W., Ste. 710
Washington, D.C. 20036
(202) 349-1155
www.lupus.org

Mary-Helen Mautner Project for Lesbians with Cancer
1707 L. Street, NW, Suite 230
Washington, DC 20036
(866) MAUTNER
www.mautnerproject.org

Muscular Dystrophy Association
National Headquarters
3300 E. Sunrise Drive
Tucson, AZ 85718
(800) 572-1717
www.mdausa.org

National Alliance for Research on Schizophrenia and Depression
60 Cutter Mill Road, Ste. 404
Great Neck, NY 11021
(800) 829-8289
narsad.org/

National Alliance on Mental Illness
Colonial Place Three
2107 Wilson Boulevard, Ste. 300
Arlington, VA 22201-3042
(888) 999-NAMI
www.nami.org

National Association for Home Care and Hospice
228 7th Street, SE
Washington, DC 20003
(202) 547-7424
www.nahc.org

National Bone Marrow Transplant Link (BMT Link)
20411 W. 12 Mile Road, Suite 108
Southfield, MI 48076
(800) LINK-BMT
www.nbmtlink.org

National Brain Tumor Foundation
22 Battery St., Ste. 612
San Francisco, CA 94111
(800) 934-CURE
www.braintumor.org

National Cancer Institute
Office of Cancer Communication
Building 31, Room 10A24
9000 Rockville Pike
Bethesda, MD 20892
(800) 4-CANCER
www.cancernet.nci.nih.gov

National Center for Complementary and Alternative Medicine
P.O. Box 7923
Gaithersburg, MD 20898-7923
(888) 644-6226
www.nccam.nih.gov

National Chronic Pain Outreach Association, Inc.
P.O. Box 274
Millboro, VA 24460
(540) 862-9437
www.chronicpain.org

National Down Syndrome Society
666 Broadway
New York, NY 10012
(800) 221-4602
info@ndss.org

National Kidney Foundation
30 E. 33rd Street, Ste. 1100
New York, NY 10016
(800) 622-9010
www.kidney.org

National Lymphedema Network
1611 Telegraph Avenue, Suite 1111
Oakland, CA 94612
(800) 541-3259
www.lymphnet.org

National Organization for Rare Disorders, Inc.
P.O. Box 1968
Danbury, CT 06813-1968
(800) 999-NORD
www.rarediseases.org

National Ovarian Cancer Coalition, Inc.
500 NE Spanish River Blvd, Suite 8
Boca Raton, FL 33431
(888) OVARIAN
www.ovarian.org

National Patient Travel Center Helpline
c/o Mercy Medical Airlift
4620 Haygood Road, Suite 1
Virginia Beach, VA 23455
(800) 296-1217
www.patienttravel.org

Oncology Nurse Society
125 Enterprise Drive
RIDC Park West
Pittsburgh, PA 15275-1214
866-257-4ONS
www.ons.org

Physician Data Query (PDQ) - see NCI
(800)- 4-CANCER (422-6237)

Post-Treatment Resource Program
215 East 68th St., Ground Floor
New York, NY 10021
www.mskcc.org

Scleroderma Foundation
12 Kent Way, Ste. 101
Byfield, MA 01922
(800) 722-HOPE
www.scleroderma.org

Skin Cancer Foundation
245 Fifth Avenue, Suite 1403
New York, NY 10016
(800) SKIN-490
www.skincancer.org

Spina Bifida Association of America
4590 MacArthur Blvd., NW, Ste. 250
Washington, DC 20007-4226
(800) 621-3141
sbaa@sbaa.org

Support for People with Oral and Head and Neck Cancer
P.O. Box 53
Locust Valley, NY 11560-0053
(800) 377-0928
www.spohnc.org

United Ostomy Association, Inc.
19772 MacArthur Boulevard, Suite 200
Irvine, CA 92612-2405
(800) 826-0826
www.uoa.org

Visiting Nurses Association of America
99 Summer St., Suite 1700
Boston, MA 02110
(800) 426-2547
www.vnaa.org

Wellness Community
919 18th Street, NW, Suite 54
Washington, DC 20006
(888) 793-WELL
www.thewellnesscommunity.org

References

1. Bertakis, K.D., Callahan, E.J., Helms, L.J., Azari, R., Robbins, J.A., and Miller, J., "Physician practice styles and patient outcomes: Differences between family practice and general internal medicine," *Medical Care* 36(6): 879–891.
2. Vilhjalmsson, R., "Direct and indirect effects of chronic physical conditions on depression: A preliminary investigation," *Social Science and Medicine.* 47(5): 603–611.
3. Watson, K., "A better argument-without getting angry," *Natural Health*, Nov-Dec, 1998.
4. Lissoni, P., Cangemi, P., Pirato, D., Roselli, M.G., Rovelli, F., Brivio, F., Malugani F., Maestroni, G.J., Conti, A., Laudon, M., Malysheva, O., and Giani, L., "A review on cancer—Psychospiritual status interactions," *Neuroendocrinology Letters* 22(3): 175–180.
5. Gruzehier, J.H., "A review of the impact of hypnosis, relaxation, guided imagery and individual differences on aspects of immunity and health," *Stress: The International Journal On the Biology of Stress* 5(2): 147-163.
6. Mundy, E.A., DuHamel, K.N., and Montgemery. G.H., "The efficacy of behavioral interventions for cancer treatment-related side effects," *Seminars in Clinical Neuropsychiatry* 8(4): 253–275.
7. Rando, T.A., *Grief, Dying and Death: Clinical Interventions for Caregivers* (Research Press Company, 1985).
8. Cathcart, C.K., Jones, S.E., Pumroy, C.S., Peters, G.N., Knox, S.M., and Cheek, J.H., "Clinical recognition and management of depression in node negative breast cancer patients treated with tamoxifen," *Breast Cancer Research & Treatment* 27(3): 277–281.
9. Curt, G.A., Breitbart, W., Cella, D., Groopman, J.E., Horning, S.J., Itri, L.M., Johnson, D.H., Miaskowski, C., Scherr, S.L., Portenoy, R.K., and Vogelzang, N.J., "Impact of cancer-related fatigue on the lives of patients: New findings from the Fatigue Coalition," *Oncologist* 5(5): 353–360.
10. Bigatti, S.M., and Cronan, T.A., "An examination of the physical health, health care use, and psychological well-being of spouses of people with fibromyalgia syndrome," Health Psychology 21(2): 157–166.
11. Morimoto, T., Schreiner, A.S., and Asano, H. "Caregiver burden and health-related quality of life among Japanese stroke survivors," Age and Aging. 32(2): 218–223.
12. Figley, C.R., ed, *Compassion Fatigue: Secondary Traumatic Stress Disorders from Treating the Traumatized* (New York: Brunner/Mazel, Inc., 1995).
13. Herbert, F., *Dune* (Philadelphia: Putnam, 1965).
14. Winston Churchill, Attributed. Quoted in *Reader's Digest*, Dec. 1954.
15. Hay, L.L., *You Can Heal Your Life* (Carlsbad, CA: Hay House, Inc., 1987), p. 219.
16. Lissoni, et al., "A review on cancer."
17. Landis, B.J., "Uncertainty, spiritual well-being, and psychosocial adjustments to chronic illness," *Issues in Mental Health Nursing* 17(3): 217–231.
18. Weiss, B.L., *Through Time into Healing* (New York: Simon & Schuster, 1992).
19. Savary, L.M., Berne, P.H., *Kything: The Art of Spiritual Presence* (Mahwah, N.J.: Paulist Press, 1988).

Bibliography

- Borysenko, J., (audio cas.), *Healing and Spirituality: The Sacred Quest for Transformation of Body and Soul.* Carlsbad, CA: Hay House, 2000.

- Jost, S., (audio cas., CDs, and book), *Cancer Involvement Program: An Integrative & Holistic Approach to Conventional Medical Treatment.* St. Louis: One Health Publishing, 2002.

- Naparstek, B., (audio cas.), *Health Journeys: A Meditation for Relaxation and Wellness.* Cleveland: Image Paths, 2002.

- Benjamin, H., *The Wellness Community Guide to Fighting for Recovery from Cancer.* New York: Putnam's Sons, 1987, 1995.

- Moore, T., *Care of the Soul.* New York: HarperCollins, 1992.

- Perls, F.S., *Gestalt Therapy Verbatim.* Moab, UT: Real People Press, 1959.

- Weiss, B., *Messages from the Masters.* New York: Warner Books, 2000.

- Zukav, G., and Francis, L., *The Heart of the Soul.* New York: Simon and Schuster, Inc., 2002.

- Hover-Kramer, D., *Healing Touch: A Guidebook for Practitioners*, 2nd Edition. New York: Delmar Books, 2002.

Index